The Origin and Evolution of Anesthesia in Japan

The Origin and Evolution of Anesthesia in Japan

By *Akitomo Matsuki*

Hirosaki University Press

Akitomo Matsuki
Emeritus Professor of Anesthesiology
Hirosaki University Graduate School of Medicine
5 Zaifu – cho, Hirosaki 036 – 8562, Japan

TITLE: The Origin and Evolution of Anesthesia in Japan

ISBN 978 – 4 – 907192 – 42 – 6

This work is subject to copyright. All rights are reserved, whether the whole or part of the material is concerned, specifically the rights of translation, reprinting, reuse of illustrations, recitation, broadcasting, reproduction on microfilms or in other ways, and storage in data banks. The use of registered names, trademarks, etc. in this publication does not imply, even in the absence of a specific statement, that such names are exempt from the relevant protective laws and regulations and therefore free for general use.

© Hirosaki University Press
First Edition, First Printing, 2017

Printed in Japan

Printing and binding: Yamato Printing Co., Ltd. Japan

The cover was designed by A. Matsuki.

Dedicated to the late Joju Takeda,
Professor of Hygiene at Hirosaki University
who warmly encouraged me to study the history of medicine
as a medical student

Contents

Preface vii

Acknowledgements ix

Explanatory Notes xi

Chapter I The Origin and Evolution of Anesthesia in Japan 1
    1 Are Historical Studies on Our Specialty Mandatory? 3
    2 Anesthesia in Japan before 1949 9
    3 Anesthesia in Japan after 1950 27
    4 The Blank 20 Years, 1925–1945 41
    5 From Historical Perspective 57

Chapter II History of Anesthesia in Japan before 1867 63
    1 Tokumei Takamine Did not Administer General Anesthetics in Ryukyu 63
    2 Hoyoku Takashi and Anesthesia–related Agents for Coaptation 71
    3 Sadakichi Iwanaga from Kyoto–Another of Hanaoka's Preceptors of Surgery 77
    4 Seishu Hanaoka's Philosophy of "Safety and Challenge" 83
    5 Introduction of Inhaled Anesthesia to Batavia and Japan 92

Chapter III History of Anesthesia in Japan between 1868 and 1949 99
    1 Otojiro Kitagawa and Spinal Morphine 99
    2 Description of Anesthesia in Japanese Textbooks of General Surgery before 1949 103
    3 Deaths due to Spinal Anesthesia in Japan before 1945 110
    4 The Blank 20 Years in the History of Anesthesia between 1925 and 1945 –The Lost 20 Years– 118
    5 Hayao Nakatani, Another Surgeon who Appreciated Modern American Anesthesiology in the 1930s 123
    6 Professor Saito, Dr. Park, and Terminal Sac Anesthesia–The First to Propose the Designation of *Saddle Block* Technique in the World in 1940– 129

Chapter IV National and International Factors that Hampered Advances in Anesthesia before the End of the Pacific War 135
    I National Factors 139
        A The Japan Surgical Society 139
            1 Japanese Allegiance to German Surgery 139
            2 Concept of "Anesthesia" among Surgeons 140

                3 A Report from Miyake's Department at Kyushu University
                   on Postoperative Mortality   141
                4 The Controversy on Thoracotomy   141
             B Japanese Medical Community   142
                1 The Japanese Association of Medical Sciences (JAMS)   142
                2 The Japan Medical Association (JMA)   142
             C The Ministry of Health and Welfare   143
             D The Ministry of Education   143
             E Pan–Asianism   143
          II International Factors   145
             A World War I   145
             B Diplomatic Problems   146
                1 Naval Reduction Conferences   146
                2 Immigration Act of 1924   146
             C Sustained Standards of German Medicine after World War I   147

Chapter V   History of Anesthesia in Japan after 1950 ·················· 153
             1 Meyer Saklad's Lectures at the JAJCME–according to Documents from
                Japanese and American Sources–   153
             2 Influence of Meyer Saklad's Lectures on Japanese Textbooks of
                Anesthesiology   158
             3 Professor Percival S. Bailey and Kentaro Shimizu –Seven Consecutive
                Chance Occurrences Leading to the Foundation of
                the First Department of Anesthesiology in Japan–   161
             4 When Did Kentaro Shimizu Determine to Establish the Department of
                Anesthesiology?   165
             5 Establishment of the First Department of Anesthesiology
                and Foundation of the Japan Society of Anesthesiology   169
             6 The First Tracheal Anesthesia for Surgery in Japan   172
             7 The Origin of "Specially Approved Designation"
                of Anesthesia and Board Certified Anesthesiologists   179
             8 Anesthesia–related Papers in the Quadrennial Meetings
                of the Japanese Association of Medical Sciences
                –Focusing on Professor Yamamura's presentations–   185

Appendix I   Revised Chronology of the History of Anesthesia in Japan ·············· 189
Appendix II   History of Anesthesia in the United States, Great Britain,
              and Other Countries ·· 213
Index of Personal Names ·· 253
Index of Subjects ·· 257

Preface

The number 60 has great significance in the Japanese culture and daily life as exemplified by the fact that we celebrate the 60th anniversary of our birth and commemorate the 60th anniversary of the foundation of any institution and company as well as the establishment of departments of universities and academic societies. In popular culture, the number 60 is believed to mean "resuscitation" or "regeneration" according to the traditional idea of combining 10 calendar signs and the 12 zodiac signs, which is originally derived from ancient China. Accordingly, the number 60 promises future development and prosperity

In 2013, we celebrated the 60th Annual Meeting of the Japanese Society of Anesthesiologists (JSA) established in 1954, with the first Annual Meeting held in the same year. The academic program committee of the JSA included several programs for its 60th annual meeting. One of them was a special lecture delivered by myself, entitled with "The Origin and Evolution of Anesthesia in Japan." The lecture aimed to provide the audience with an outline of the history of anesthesiology in Japan and provide a perspective of the specialty that I considered indispensable as we looked back at the history of our specialty while on the edge of "regeneration." I also provided my thoughts on where we were from and where we were going to.

Chapter Ⅰ of this book is a reproduction of the lecture that I delivered at the 60th Annual Meeting of the JSA, with all slides that I used at the lecture reproduced with corresponding explanations and references. By employing this method, although quite different from conventional editing style, I am convinced that this approach will allow readers to understand my lectures more deeply than from explanations without slides. The lecture was a concise history of anesthesia in Japan since the beginning of the 19th century, when, in October 1804, Seishu Hanaoka gave an oral anesthetic "Mafutsusan" to a 60-year-old woman, Kan Aiya, for excision of her breast cancer tumor, up to the latest event in 2011 when the Japanese Museum of Anesthesiology was founded in Kobe.

In the Chapters Ⅱ–Ⅴ, significant events, episodes, and their backgrounds are described in detail to provide a further description of the history of anesthesia in Japan according to my proposed period divisions: prior to 1867; between 1868 and 1949; and after 1950. A special emphasis on the period "between 1868 and 1949," as in Chapter IV of the "National and International Factors that Hampered Advances in Anesthesia before the End of the Pacific War," is provided because advances in the specialty decreased during this period for previously undefined reasons. The majority of members of the JSA assumed that the Pacific War was the only cause of the hampered advances in anesthesiology before the war in Japan. Chapter IV was thus included to dispel this widely disseminated misapprehension among JSA members.

The "Revised chronology of the History of Anesthesia in Japan" in Appendix I provides a brief overview of the history of our specialty and offers suggestions for future studies in this field. The papers in Appendix II commemorate Professor Elemér K. Zsigmond, who was generous in allowing me the chance to conduct historical studies of anesthesiology during my visit to the University of Michigan. Despite these studies being reported several decades ago, I believe many of them remain relevant to the field of anesthesiology today.

January 2017

Akitomo Matsuki

Acknowledgements

I am grateful to Emeritus Professor Hideo Yamamura from the Department of Anesthesiology at the University of Tokyo Graduate School of Medicine for his invaluable advice and continuous encouragement. I express my cordial appreciation to Hisayo O. Morishima, Emeritus Professor from the Department of Anesthesiology and Obstetrics/Gynecology, College of Physicians and Surgeons at Columbia University, for her valuable suggestions and encouragement. I would like to thank Dr. Kazuyoshi Hirota, Professor and Chairman, Department of Anesthesiology, Hirosaki University Graduate School of Medicine and Dr. Hironori Ishihara, the director of Kuroishi Kosei Hospital, for providing insightful comments.

I express my cordial thanks to Dr. Tomoko Takazawa, one of my professional colleagues and classmate at medical school, for her ongoing encouragement in my study of the history of anesthesiology.

I would like to extend my deepest gratitude to Ms. Yuki Narita from the Hirosaki University Press for her editorial advice and Mrs. Kou Mikami and Mrs. Miyuki Fukuyama, secretaries of the Department of Anesthesiology at Hirosaki University Graduate School of Medicine for their assistance.

I am grateful to the following people for giving me permission to reproduce the photographs and illustrations, appearing in this book:

Persons (in alphabetical order)
Koji Takamine for Figure 2.1.1 and Figure 2.1.2.
Hitoshi Matsunaga for Figure5.6.1, Figure5.6.3–6, and Figure5.6.10.

Institutions (in alphabetical order)
Kyoto University for Figure 2.3.2.
Kyo–u Library for Figure 2.3.3 and Figure 2.3.4.
Sendai Museum for Figure 2.1.3 and Figure 2.1.4.
University of Tokyo Library for Figure 2.5.1.

Explanatory Notes

1. References and Remarks were shown in the end of each section for readers' convenience.

2. Names of books, journals, and manuscripts were expressed in italics.

3. The terms "anesthesia" and "anesthesiology," "local anesthesia" and "regional anesthesia," and "endotracheal anesthesia" and "tracheal anesthesia" were used interchangeably.

4. The lunar calendar was used for Japanese events before December 3, 1872.

Chapter I The Origin and Evolution of Anesthesia in Japan

This chapter is an English translation of a special lecture that I delivered in May 2013 at the 60th Annual Meeting of the Japanese Society of Anesthesiologists (JSA) in Sapporo, Japan.[1,2] Although the original lecture comprised 50 slides, 10 further slides have been added in this chapter to make the lecture more accurate, understandable, and up-to-date. In some of the 50 slides and their explanations, minor but necessary revisions have been made to acquaint readers with advances in the field that have occurred in the 3 years subsequent to the lecture.

The 50 slides were initially in Japanese; however, they were also translated into English. In this chapter, for the convenience of readers, two slides are presented on each left-hand page (verso), and their explanations are transcribed on the facing page (recto). References and remarks are also shown at the bottom of the explanatory pages for the convenience of readers. In the explanations, the word "anesthesia" is used to mean both "anesthesia" and "anesthesiology." In addition, the term "local anesthesia" is employed to mean both "local anesthesia" and "regional anesthesia."

The lecture is a concise and comprehensive review of the 200-year history of anesthesia in Japan. For readers interested in further information on the topics covered in this lecture, a more detailed background and discussion of these topics are provided in Chapter II, III, IV, and V.

1. Matsuki A. The Origin and Evolution of Anesthesia in Japan. *Masui* 2013; 62: S1–S10.
2. Matsuki A. *Unknown Episodes in the History of Anesthesia in Japan* (*Postwar period*). Tokyo, Shinkokoeki Ishoshuppanbu, 2014. p.13–80.

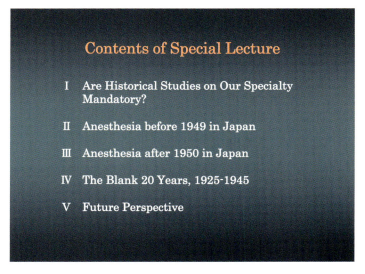

Slide 1

Slide 3

1 Are Historical Studies on Our Specialty Mandatory?

Slide 1   It is a great honor for me to deliver this special lecture on the occasion of the 60th Annual Meeting of the JSA in Sapporo, Japan. First, I would like to express my thanks to Professor Hiroshi Iwasaki of Asahikawa Medical University, Asahikawa, Japan, president of this annual meeting, for inviting me to give this special lecture. Second, I would like to extend my deep appreciation to Professor Kiyoshi Morita of Okayama University, Okayama, Japan, for his chairmanship of this lecture. Finally, I would like to express my gratitude to the Scientific Program Committee members for their diligent organization.

The number 60 has a special significance in the Japanese manner of thinking. We celebrate our 60th birthday as an auspicious felicity because it represents the regeneration of life according to the sexagenary cycle. Accordingly, I think that the 60th anniversary of the JSA is an excellent occasion on which we can express our profound appreciation to the pioneers who founded our society and assiduously devoted themselves to its development. It is also an unequaled opportunity for us to examine the present status of the society by reflecting on its past and contemplating its future.

Slide 2   Declaration of interest   None declared.

Slide 3   As shown in this slide, the lecture consists of five chapters. In the first chapter, the significance and importance of historical studies are discussed. To be an excellent teacher of medical care related to anesthesia, it is appropriate, if not mandatory, to be acquainted with the history of the field. In the second chapter, I relate the history of anesthesia in Japan before 1949, and in the third chapter, I describe the progress in our specialty after 1950. This distinction is made because in 1950, Meyer Saklad (1901–1979) visited Japan as a member of the Unitarian Service Committee Medical Mission to introduce the modern American practice of anesthesia. His lectures made an enormous impact on Japanese professors of surgery, who were unfamiliar even with the term "anesthesiology" as a clinical discipline. Thus, 1950 is a particularly significant year in our history.

In the 75 years between 1870 and 1945, Japanese medicine was exclusively influenced by the German style of medicine. In 1875, the Meiji Government adopted the German model of medical care and education. Subsequently, Japanese physicians neglected American and British medical practices because these styles were ranked secondary to that of Germany. The reasons why we overlooked their styles of medical practice are discussed in detail in the fourth chapter, entitled "The Blank 20 Years, 1925–1945."[1] In the fifth and last chapter, I describe the future perspectives of our society.

1. It was originally "The Blank 21 Years, 1924–1945," and revised to "The Blank 20 Years, 1925–1945." See Slides 40 and 55.

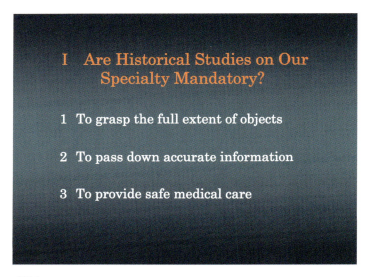

Slide 4

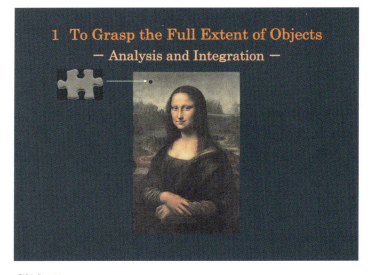

Slide 5

Slide 4   I think that it is important to be acquainted with the history of a discipline because it is impossible to appreciate its essence without knowledge of its history and development. We must not ignore important discoveries by our antecedents. In an epistle[1] to Robert Hooke (1635–1703) in 1675, Isaac Newton (1642–1727) wrote, "If I have seen further it is by standing on the shoulders of giants."[2] In this phrase, when saying "the shoulders of giants," Newton is referring to the significant discoveries of past pioneers. Therefore, it is vital to understand the importance of past discoveries and related historical studies. As shown in this slide, the importance comprises three parts. They are as follows:

1. to grasp the full extent of objects or events;
2. to pass down accurate information on the histories of objects or events to the next generation; and
3. to provide safer medical care to patients.

Slide 5   One of the purposes of a historical study is to grasp the full extent of an object. Science is used to analyze the object and elucidate and describe its mechanism. However, we are unable to gain an overall perspective of the object by analysis alone, and we must integrate the analyzed parts of the object to reveal the whole picture. This slide shows a jigsaw puzzle, symbolizing the relationship between analysis (many pieces) and integration (the complete picture; for example, the Mona Lisa by Leonardo Da Vinci). A profound appreciation of an object can only be obtained through a historical approach because these historical studies allow integration. Consequently, science requires both analysis and integration, and historical perspectives are indispensable for such integration.

1. The epistle was dated February 5, 1675.
2. Turnbull HW. ed. *The Correspondence of Isaac Newton.* (Vol.1) Cambridge, Cambridge University Press, 1959. p.416–7.

2 To Pass Down Accurate Information

Major innovations were sometimes ignored until their rediscovery several decades later.

Larson, M.D. : History of Anesthetic Practice. *Miller's Anesthesia.* 7th ed., 2010. p.3

Slide 6

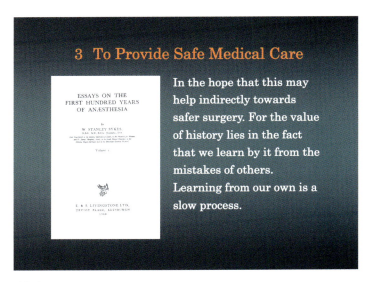

3 To Provide Safe Medical Care

In the hope that this may help indirectly towards safer surgery. For the value of history lies in the fact that we learn by it from the mistakes of others.
Learning from our own is a slow process.

Slide 7

Slide 6   As shown in this slide, Merlin D. Larson(1931–), a professor of anesthesiology at the University of California at San Francisco in the United States, emphasized that historical studies can unfold overlooked discoveries in our specialty.[1] Many historical facts remain unknown, and from this situation, ambiguous stories can arise, leading to misconceptions. We are unable to draw useful conclusions to present to subsequent generations from erroneous records.

Slide 7   Historical approaches are also mandatory for providing safer medical care to patients. Safety standards in current medical practice are the results of accidents and incidents in the past. Therefore, we must learn from these mistakes through historical studies. As shown in this slide, these few sentences taken from the dedication in W. Stanley Sykes' (1894–1961) book[2] describe the loss of his father, who underwent cholecystectomy and died thereafter. The subsequent loss of his father–in–law, who underwent the same procedure and ultimately experienced the same fate, is also described therein. These tragedies demonstrate a failure to learn from prior mistakes. I often repeat Sykes' phrases during my lectures, and some of you may be familiar with them; however, I entreat you again to appreciate Sykes' words.

1. Larson MD. History of Anesthetic Practice. In Miller RD. ed. *Miller's Anesthesia*. (7th ed. Vol.1) Philadelphia, Churchill Livingstone, 2010. p.3–41.
2. Sykes SW. *Essays on The First Hundred Years of Anaesthesia*. (Vol. 1) Edinburgh, E. & S. Livingstone, 1960. Dedication.

8　Chapter I　The Origin and Evolution of Anesthesia in Japan

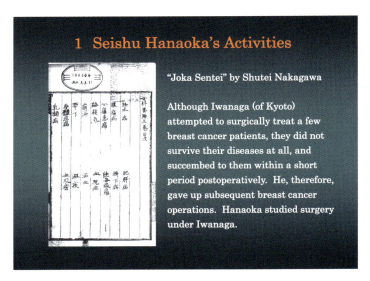

Slide 8

Slide 9

2 Anesthesia in Japan before 1949

Slide 8   I will now move on to the second chapter, in which I present the history of anesthesia in Japan before 1949. The chapter is divided into the following four sections:

1. the role of Seishu Hanaoka's activities;
2. the introduction of inhalation anesthesia by Seikei Sugita;
3. the tuition of Japanese surgeons in German-speaking countries in the Meiji era; and
4. anesthesia in Japan before the end of the Pacific War.

Slide 9   Seishu Hanaoka (1760–1835) is the greatest pioneer in the history of anesthesia in the Edo period in Japan. Although many articles have been written on his life and work, some contain erroneous information. I would like to introduce you the most recent and correct information. This slide shows a manuscript, entitled "*Joka Sentei*" (*Introduction to Woman's Diseases*) by Shutei Nakagawa (1771–1850), a close and junior colleague of Hanaoka. In the manuscript, Nakagawa says the following:

> "Although Iwanaga of Kyoto attempted to surgically treat a few breast cancer patients, they did not survive their diseases at all and succumbed to them within a short period postoperatively. He therefore gave up subsequent breast cancer operations. Hanaoka studied surgery under Iwanaga."

The manuscript conveys new and significant information, for example, elucidating that Iwanaga performed breast cancer surgeries before Hanaoka, supposedly under general anesthesia achieved with an anesthetic concoction mainly consisting of Datura. Although details of the patients, anesthetic methods used, and the exact dates of the operations are unclear, it is apparent that Iwanaga attempted breast cancer surgery before Hanaoka's successful procedure in 1804. According to my recent study,[1] Iwanaga was likely to be a second generation member of the Iwanaga family of Kyoto, who practiced the Dutch style of surgery. Hanaoka's father Naomichi was also a Dutch style surgeon and a disciple of a surgeon named Juseki Iwanaga, who was a second-generation member of the Iwanaga family from Osaka.

1. Matsuki A. *New Development in the Study of Seishu Hanaoka*. Tokyo, Shinkokoeki Ishoshuppanbu, 2013. p.99–108.

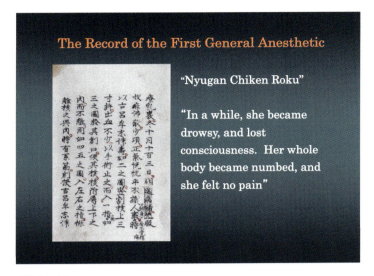

Slide 10

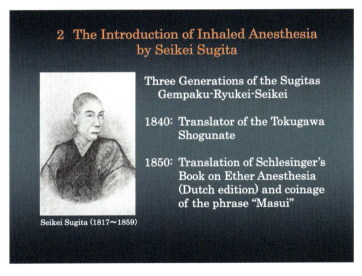

Slide 11

Slide 10   To completely understand the background of the administration of the first general anesthetic by Hanaoka, we must also discuss another important issue. In October 1804, for the first time, Hanaoka administered "Mafutsusan," an oral general anesthetic, to a woman named Kan Aiya (1745–1805) for the excision of a breast cancer tumor. The case is described in the manuscript *Nyugan Chiken Roku*" as shown on the left–hand side of this slide. The presence of several erroneous Chinese characters with the same pronunciation in the sentences suggests that it may have been recorded from Hanaoka's dictation by one of his disciples. Hanaoka used 17 Chinese characters to describe the physical state of Kan (shown on the right–hand side of the slide), who lost sensation and consciousness after taking "Mafutsusan."[1] If he had a well–defined idea of general anesthesia, he could have described her condition in two to four Chinese characters. Ryukei Sugita (1786–1845), to whom Hanaoka disclosed the formula of the drug and how to administer it, used only two Chinese characters, "*Ma*" and "*Sui*," to express the loss of sensation and awareness induced by the anesthetic, although he employed a different Chinese character, "*Sui*," with the same sound.

Hanaoka's goal was to surgically treat women with breast cancer, and to achieve his purpose he finally developed a concoction that produced general anesthesia during operations, preventing both consciousness and pain. Although he was unlikely to be primarily concerned with how to express the state produced by the agent in Chinese characters, this does nothing to discredit him as the pioneer of anesthesia in Japan.

Slide 11   Hanaoka's method of anesthesia using "Mafutsusan" was frequently and widely used by many disciples throughout the country; however, its use gradually declined toward the end of the Tokugawa period and Meiji era for several reasons, including Hanaoka's death in 1835, his successor Shuhei's death in 1866, and the prolonged induction and delayed recovery intrinsic to the method. In addition, information on inhalational anesthesia using ether and chloroform from the Netherlands was introduced in the 1850s and 1860s. Shown in this slide, Seikei Sugita (1817–1859) was a grandson of Gempaku Sugita (1733–1817), famous for the translation of *Kaitai Shinsho* in 1774, and a son of Ryukei Sugita, mentioned in the previous slide. Seikei was a formal translator for the Tokugawa shogunate and translated a Dutch edition of J. Schlesinger's German textbook of ether anesthesia in 1850. He coined the phrase "Masui" using the same two Chinese characters we use today.[2]

1. Matsuki A. *New Development in the Study of Seishu Hanaoka*. p.132–6.
2. Matsuki A. *A Short History of Anesthesia in Japan*. Hirosaki, Hirosaki University Press, 2012. p.78–80.

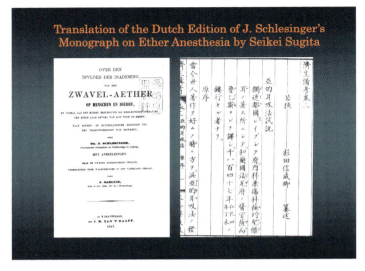

Slide 12

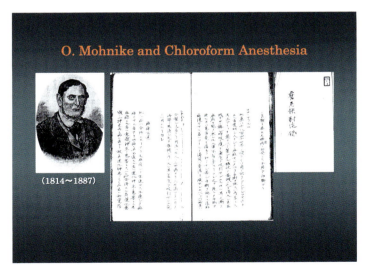

Slide 13

Slide 12   On the left-hand side of the slide, the title page of the Dutch edition of J. Schlesinger's textbook of 1847[1] is shown, which is entitled *Over den Invloed der Inademing van den Zwavel–Aether op Menschen en Dieren* (*On the Effects of Inhalation of Sulfuric Ether on Men and Animals*), and the right-hand side of the slide shows the title page of the Japanese translation by Seikei Sugita, entitled *Ateru Kyuho Shisetsu*, (*Treatise on the Inhalation of Ether*), which was published in 1850.

Slide 13   The left-hand side of the slide shows a portrait of the Dutch physician Otto Mohnike (1814–1887), and the right-hand side depicts the manuscript, entitled "*A Dialogue with Mohnike*," by the Japanese physician Soken Narabayashi (1802–1852) of the Saga Domain. Mohnike visited Japan in June 1848 as a medical attaché to the Dutch East India Company factory at Dejima in Nagasaki, Japan.[1] Two months later, he informed Narabayashi of chloroform analgesia, which Narabayashi recorded in the manuscript.[2] In June 1849, a Dutch copy of Schlesinger's book on ether anesthesia was imported to Japan and its Japanese translation by Seikei Sugita was published in March 1850. In August 1851, Mohnike talked of ether anesthesia with Shinsuke Maeda (1821–1901), a physician from the Kagoshima Domain, relating that ether was ineffective as a general anesthetic and delayed postoperative wound healing and that it was therefore never employed in Western countries.

It is a strange and inconsistent story: chloroform anesthesia was discovered in 1847 and information about it was brought to Japan in 1848, whereas ether anesthesia was discovered in 1846, and information about it arrived in Japan in 1849. The use of ether anesthesia preceded that of chloroform anesthesia worldwide, with Japan being the only exception. This discrepancy was caused by Mohnike's deliberate neglect of ether anesthesia because he inappropriately considered it to be ineffective and detrimental.

1. Matsuki A. *A Short History of Anesthesia in Japan*. p.81–4.
2. ibid. p.73–8.

Chapter I The Origin and Evolution of Anesthesia in Japan

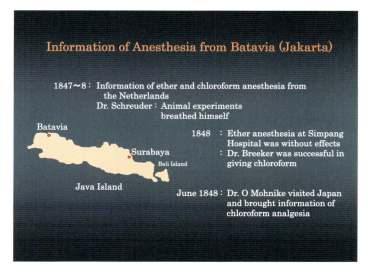

Slide 14

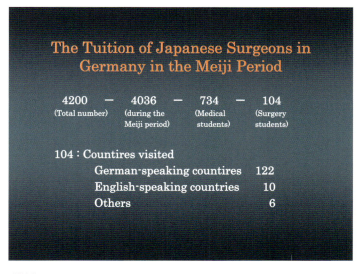

Slide 15

Slide 14   Why Mohnike recommended chloroform but not ether to Narabayashi can be explained by the practice of anesthesia at the time in Batavia (present–day Jakarta, Indonesia), the capital of Dutch East India, where the government ran several hospitals. The physicians, Mohnike among them, were from the Netherlands. During the years 1847–1848, ether and then chloroform were introduced to Batavia. Initially, physicians experimented with ether to observe its anesthetic effects on frogs, mice, and dogs, and then studied its effects on strychnine–induced intoxication in dogs. A physician Schreuder himself tried twice to inhale the agent for approximately 30 min, causing only headache and dizziness without expected effects. At the Simpang Hospital in Surabaya, Dutch East India, another physician Wassink administered the drug to seven surgical patients, but was unsuccessful in providing them with adequate clinical anesthesia. In early 1848, chloroform was introduced, and four leg amputations were performed by Drs. Bleeker and Wassink using the agent. Although the anesthesia was incomplete, patients' complaints were "nothing compared with the screams that were formerly heard in similar cases."[1] Therefore, it is apparent that Mohnike observed and realized the inefficacy of ether and efficacy of chloroform before he visited Japan. This is the most likely reason why he intentionally neglected ether anesthesia and only focused on chloroform anesthesia when talking to Narabayashi.

Slide 15   Although the Tokugawa shogunate closed the country in 1633, Western– style medicine was uninterruptedly brought by Dutch and German physicians of the Dutch East India Company factory in Dejima, Nagasaki for the subsequent two and a half centuries. However, the modality by which Western medicine was introduced into our country dramatically changed at the very end of the Edo period (1861–1867) and start of the Meiji era (1868–1912), when Japanese students began studying abroad. This slide shows the number of students who studied abroad. At the end of the Edo period and start of the Meiji era, 4200 public and private students of liberal and scientific disciplines studied abroad, whereas 4036 students studied in the Meiji era. Of these 4036 students, 734 were medical students, 104 of which were surgery students. Among them, 122 students visited German–speaking countries, 10 visited English–speaking countries, and six visited other countries. Some traveled to two or more countries; therefore, the total number (138) of surgery students according to the countries they visited is higher than the actual number (104).[2]

1. Schoute D. *Occidental therapeutics in the Netherlands East Indies during three Centuries of Netherlands Settlement.* (*1600–1900*). Batavia, G. Kolff, 1937. p.147.
2. The data are based on the following book.
   Tezuka A. and National Education Center. eds. *A Conspectus of Japanese Student who studied abroad in the End of the Edo Period and the Meiji era*. Tokyo, Kashiwa Shobo, 1992.

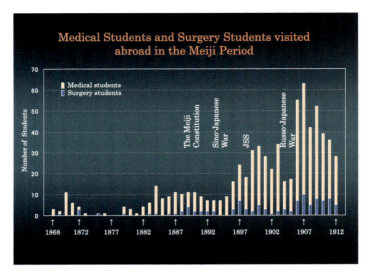

Slide 16

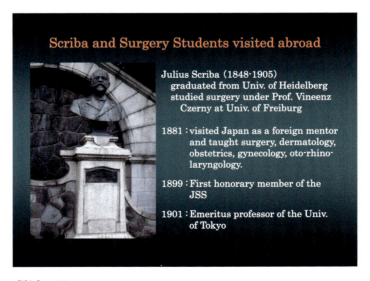

Slide 17

Slide 16   This slide illustrates the annual number of medical students who studied abroad during the Meiji era. Yellow columns indicate medical students and blue columns indicate surgical students. Four peaks are present among the columns. The first small peak represents the period 1868–1872, suggesting that our government sent a few competent medical students abroad for the urgent purpose of establishing medical research and a medical education system in Japan. The second peak represents the period 1884–1892, corresponding to a period of maturation of the nation's governmental system, as supported by the promulgation of the Meiji Constitution (1889). The third peak represents the period 1896–1903, which coincides with the period after the Sino–Japanese War (1894–1895). The fourth and largest peak represents the period 1906–1912, followed by the Russo–Japanese War (1904–1905). In general, surgical students mainly studied in German–speaking countries in the period 1880–1910.

Slide 17   As mentioned earlier, the Meiji Government adopted the German system of medical care and education and invited physicians from Germany. Julius Scriba (1848–1905) was the most influential surgeon among them. As shown in this slide, he graduated from the University of Heidelberg, Germany, and he then moved to the University of Freiburg, Germany, where he was a lecturer under Professor Vincenz Czerny (1842–1916). He relocated to study surgery further under Professor Bernard von Langenbeck (1810–1887) at the University of Berlin. In 1881, the University of Tokyo invited him to act as a foreign mentor of surgery, where he taught surgery, dermatology, obstetrics, ophthalmology, and otorhinolaryngology, and trained many students in surgery and other specialties. Almost all professors of surgery in Japan in the Meiji era were Scriba's disciples. Because of his enormous contribution to the Japanese surgery, he was granted the title of the first honorary member of the Japan Surgical Society (JSS), when the first annual meeting of the society was held in Tokyo in 1899.[1,2] Consequently, most of the Japanese medical students trained by him studied abroad in his native country or German–speaking countries.

1. Anonym. Julius Scriba, The First Honorary Member. *J. Japan Surgical Society.* 2000; 101 (Supplement): 31.
2. Kanbara H. A Pre-history of the Japanese Orthopaedic Association. In Tajima T. ed. *60 Years' Progress of The Japanese Orthopaedic Association in Commemoration of its 60th Annual Meeting.* Niigata, Editorial Board of 60 Years' Progress of The Japanese Orthopaedic Association in Commemoration of its 60th Annual Meeting. Department of Orthopedic Surgery, Niigata University School of Medicine, 1987. p.5–6.

Several Important Discoveries in German Anesthesia in 1884-1910

Year	Person	Discovery
1884	Carl Koller	discovers clinical use of cocaine
1890	P.Vera Redard	introduces the ethyl chloride spray for local anesthesia
1891	Ferdinand Giesel	discovers and isolates tropacocaine
1891	Heinrich Quincke	discovers the clinical use of lumbar puncture
1892	Carl L Schreich	discovers local infiltration anesthesia
1895	Alfred Kirstein	introduces tracheal tubes via the first direct-vision laryngoscope
1897	Heinrich Braun	advocates the addition of epinephrine to cocaine solution
1898	August Bier	practices the first successful use of spinal anesthesia
1903	Emil Fisher	synthesizes an intravenous agent veronal
1904	Alfred Einhorn	discovers novocaine
1905	Heinrich Braun	develops the clinical use of novocaine
1905	Heinrich Braun	publishes *Die Lokalanaesthesie*
1907	Erwin Payr	develops the clinical use of eucaine
1908	August Bier	discovers intravenous regional anesthesia
1910	R Kümmell	practices the first successful use of intravenous hedonal

Slide 18

Foundation of the Japan Surgical Society (JSS)

1896 : Harutoyo Omori
       Sankichi Sato
       Yoshinori Tashiro   plan to found JSS

1898 : JSS founded

1899 : First Annual Meeting of JSS
       (President Sankichi Sato)

1872 : Deutsche Gesellschaft für Chirurgie
       Archiv für klinische Chirurgie
       (Bernhard von Langenbeck)

Slide 19

Slide 18   During the period 1884–1910, several important discoveries were made in the specialty of anesthesia, particularly related to local anesthesia, in German–speaking countries. This slide shows some of these discoveries, and it is clear that the incredible contribution these countries made to establish the basis of local and regional anesthesia. As I mentioned earlier, many Japanese surgery students studied in these countries in this period, suggesting that they gained an appreciation of the importance of local anesthesia for pain relief during surgical procedures.[1,2]

Slide 19   In 1896, several eminent surgeons, including Harutoyo Omori (1852–1912) of the Fukuoka Medical School, Fukuoka, Japan, Sankichi Sato (1857–1943) and Yoshinori Tashiro (1864–1938) of the University of Tokyo, started discussing the possibility of establishing an academic society in which they could read their papers and exchange their opinions. Their founding plan for the society must have been much encouraged by the great efforts of Professor Bernhard von Langenbeck, who started publishing the *Archives of Clinical Surgery* in 1860 and founded the German Society of Surgery in 1872.[3]

In November, 1898, they formulated a draft of the society's rules and the JSS was established. In April 1899, the first annual meeting was held in Tokyo under the presidency of Sato.

1. Keys TE. *The History of Surgical Anesthesia*. New York, Schuman's, 1945.
2. Rushman GB, Davies NJH, and Atkinson RS. *A Short History of Anaesthesia. The first 150 Years*. Oxford, Butterworth –Heinemann, 1996.
3. Rutkow IM. *Surgery An Illustrated History*. St Louis, Mosby, 1993. p.393.

20 Chapter I The Origin and Evolution of Anesthesia in Japan

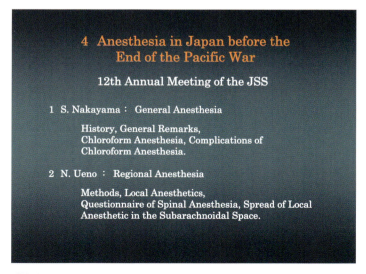

Slide 20

Slide 21

Slide 20   This slide contains a list of the first to 30th presidents of the annual meetings of the JSS. All except Kanehiro Takaki, the fourth president, studied in German–speaking countries, and their periods of study extended from 1869 to 1917. Japanese surgery achieved rapid progress under the leadership of these eminent surgeons who studied in these countries, indicating that the system of patient care, education, and research in Japan was under the dominant influence of the German model. Consequently, as far as the practice of anesthesia was concerned, it is reasonable to suppose that Japanese surgeons at that time placed a higher priority on local anesthesia than on general anesthesia.

Slide 21   In Japan, the practice of anesthesia had not been significantly evaluated in the clinical setting. This is supported by the following fact: "Anesthesia" was chosen as the main theme on only a single occasion at the 50 annual meetings of the JSS between 1899 and 1949. On this occasion in 1911, special reports on general and local anesthesia were presented by Shigeki Nakayama (1879–1962?)[1] and Nobushiro Ueno (1872–1932)[2]. Japanese surgeons neglected remarkable advances in the field made in the United States and United Kingdom in the corresponding period. "Tracheal Anesthesia" should at least have been a theme for discussion during meetings in 1920s and 1930s. Generally speaking, Japanese surgeons at that time considered anesthesia an expedient for accommodating the operator alone.

1. Nakayama S. General anesthesia. *J. Japan Surgical Society* 1911; 12: 177–304.
2. Ueno N. Local anesthesia. *J. Japan Surgical Society* 1911; 12: 305–38.

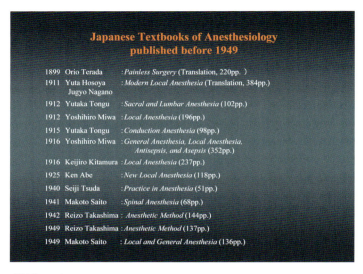

Slide 22

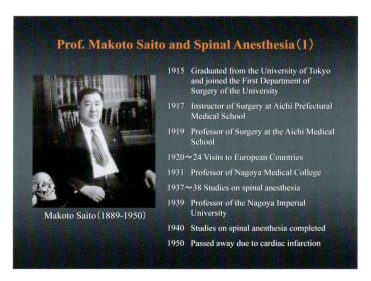

Slide 23

Slide 22 Before the end of the Pacific War in 1945, Japanese surgeons tended to opt for the use of local anesthesia over the use of general anesthesia because they considered local anesthesia to be much safer. This is substantiated by the number of textbooks on local anesthesia published at that time.[1] This slide contains a list of textbooks on anesthesia published before 1949 in Japan. As shown in this slide, 13 books were published. Takashima's book of 1949 was almost the same as his book of 1942. Although slight revisions were made in the 1949 edition, the latter can be excluded from the discussion. Eight of the remaining 12 textbooks (66.7%) are exclusively devoted to local anesthesia, and most are Japanese translations of German textbooks or abstracts from them. The remaining four cover general and local anesthesia. Among them, the most systematic description is found in Miwa's textbook, however, it is not an independent monograph but one of a series of surgical textbooks.

Slide 23 Among the studies on anesthesia conducted in Japan before the end of the Pacific War, Professor Saito's study on spinal anesthesia using a hyperbaric solution is considered of special significance. In this slide, a short biography of Saito is presented. He was a pioneer in neurosurgery in Japan. In 1937, he underwent an appendectomy under spinal anesthesia using a hypobaric solution of pantocaine (tetracaine); however, the level of anesthesia extended to the lower cervical dermatomes as a result of cephalad migration of the agent in the spinal column.[2,3] Although he developed dyspnea and dysphonia, he fortunately recovered from these complications uneventfully. Subsequently, he pledged to develop a safer method of spinal anesthesia.

1. Matsuki A. *The Origin of Anesthesiology, continued.* Tokyo, Shinkokoeki Ishoshuppanbu, 2009. p.253–95.
2. *Saito M. Local Anesthesia and General Anesthesia.* Tokyo, Gakujutsu Shoin, 1949. p.49.
3. Matsuki A. ed. *Professor Saito and Spinal Anesthesia.* Hirosaki, Private Edition, 2000. p.17–22.

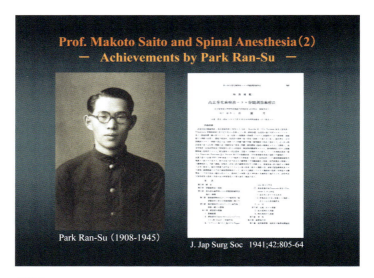

Slide 24

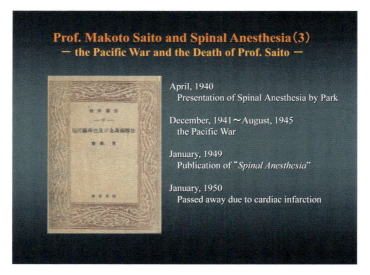

Slide 25

Slide 24   Saito recruited Park, a young Korean member of Saito's department who joined in 1936 to study surgery. In the left–hand side of the slide, a photograph of Park taken in approximately 1935–1936 is shown. Park was an excellent and hard–working researcher who was ingenious in experiments and careful in clinical work.[1] Using a glass model of the human spinal column, he identified that a hyperbaric solution with 5 –10% glucose was the best choice for spinal anesthesia. He successfully used the method on approximately 360 patients and presented his paper at the annual meeting of the JSS in 1940, which attracted the attention of every surgeon. The paper appeared in the society's journal the following year, as depicted on the right–hand side of the slide.

Slide 25   Saito and Park were eager to publicize their new method of spinal anesthesia using a hyperbaric solution; however, just 4 months after Park's paper appeared in the society's journal, the Pacific War broke out. Naturally, surgeons' concerns were not focused on this newly devised technique of spinal anesthesia, and Saito's method was not disseminated as widely as Saito intended. In 1949, 4 years after the end of the war, Saito published a booklet on anesthesia illustrated in the slide,[2] which included the essentials of the method that he intended to disseminate. However, he died the following year due to a cardiac infarction. His booklet was thus neglected.

Over the decades that followed the end of the war, many fatal spinal accidents were reported. These tragedies may have resulted from surgeons' immature understanding of spinal anesthesia, partly through their neglect of Saito's booklet which described the essence to regulate the levels of anesthesia, and partly because former military surgeons, who had been inadequately trained because of the war, returned to Japan from the front and practiced spinal anesthesia.

1. Matsuki A. ed. *Professor Saito and Spinal Anesthesia*. p.29–36.
2. Saito's booklet was reproduced in Matsuki's *Professor Saito and Spinal Anesthesia*. with annotations. (p. 57–333)

26 Chapter I The Origin and Evolution of Anesthesia in Japan

III Anesthesia after 1950 in Japan

1. American Medical Missions in 1950, 1951, and 1956
2. Establishment of Independent Department and Foundation of Japanese Society of Anesthesiology
3. Governmental Approval of Specialty and Qualification System
4. 5th World Congress of Anaesthesiologists

Slide 26

1 Medical Missions to Japan

August 1945	: the Pacific War ended
July 1950	: 1st Medical Mission (Dr. M. Saklad)
April 1951	: 51st Annual Meeting of the JSS (Maeda's Presidential Lecture)
July 1952	: 2nd Medical Mission (Prof. P. Volpitto)
July 1952	: Department of Anesthesiology is established at the Univ. of Tokyo
May 1954	: Foundation of Japanese Society of Anesthesiology
April 1956	: 3rd Medical Mission (Assoc. Prof. J.F. Artusio, Jr.)

Slide 27

3   Anesthesia in Japan after 1950

Slide 26   I will now move to the third chapter, in which I present the history of anesthesia after 1950. As shown in this slide, the four topics constituting this chapter are are as follows:

1. visits by American medical missions to Japan;
2. establishment of an independent department of anesthesia and the foundation of the JSA;
3. governmental approval of the specialty and qualification system; and
4. the fifth World Congress of Anaesthesiologists (WCA) in 1972.

Slide 27   Several years after the end of the war, the General Headquarters of the Allied Powers (GHQ) realized that the Japanese medical system was behind the times with regard to patient care and student education and should be urgently improved.

As shown in this slide, to achieve this, they dispatched medical missions to Japan in 1950, 1951, and 1956 with the cooperation of the Unitarian Service Committee.[1-4] The missions had a great impact on every field of basic and clinical medical sciences and, most remarkably, on the specialty of anesthesia, as supported by the fact that the first independent department of anesthesia was established at the University of Tokyo in 1952 and the JSA was founded in 1954, both of which occurred within a few years of the visits of the first and second missions. The first mission of the three made the greatest contribution to the history of our specialty.

1. Matsuki A. *A Short History of Anesthesia in Japan*. p.161–9.
2. Matsuki A. *The Acceptance of Anesthesiology and its Development in Japan*. Tokyo, Shinkokoeki Ishoshuppanbu, 2011. p.228–37.
3. Ikeda S. The Unitarian Service Committee Medical Mission. *Anesthesiology*. 2007; 106: 178–85.
4. Ikeda S. American anesthesiologists' contribution to post–World War II global anesthesiology: the Unitarian Service Committee's medical missions. *J. Clinical Anesthesia* 2011; 23: 244–52.

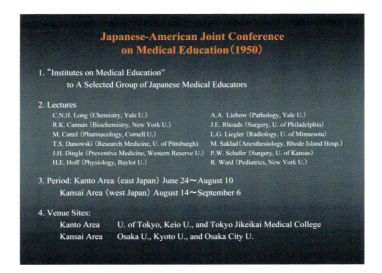

Slide 28

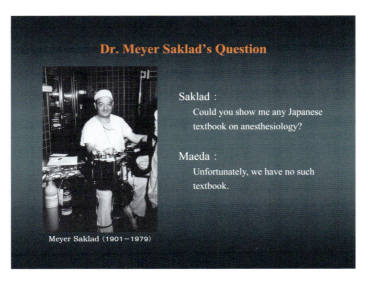

Slide 29

Slide 28   This slide provides an outline of the first medical mission in 1950. You may remember Professor S. Ikeda's (1937–) lecture given at the JSA meeting in 2012 on medical missions from the United States and the institutes they provided.[1] Japanese professors of basic and clinical medical sciences were forced to receive lectures on their own specialties at these institutes, and the most significant lectures were given by Meyer Saklad (1901–1979), a member of the first mission and the chief of the Department of Anesthesia at the Rhode Island Hospital, Providence in the United States. This was because the difference in academic standards between Japan and the United States was much more pronounced in the specialty of anesthesia than in any other discipline, including basic and clinical medical sciences.

Slide 29   Saklad, shown on the left–hand side of the slide, visited Wasaburo Maeda (1894–1979), a professor of surgery at Keio University, Tokyo, and the Japanese mediator of surgery and anesthesia sessions at the institute. When Saklad met him in his office for a preliminary discussion, his first question to Maeda was "Could you show me any Japanese textbook on anesthesiology?" Maeda answered, "Unfortunately, we have no such textbook."

1. Ikeda S. American contributions to Japanese anesthesiology – a Historical Review –. *Masui* 2013; 62: 761–9.

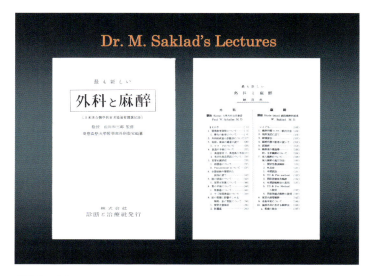

Slide 30

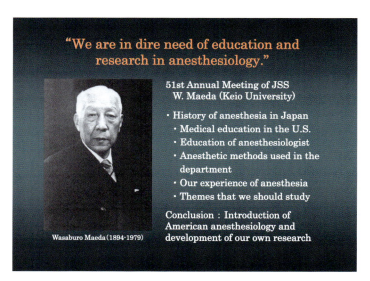

Slide 31

Slide 30   Maeda published the proceedings of surgery and anesthesia sessions at the institute only 4 months later in January 1951.[1] It contained Paul W. Schafer's lectures on medical education and surgery and Meyer Saklad's lectures on anesthesia. At the institute, various lectures were given at basic medical and clinical sessions; however, no proceedings were edited for publication, except for Maeda's. With regard to the conversation between Saklad and Maeda, it must have been a bitter experience for Maeda, and it seems likely to have galvanized him to publish the proceedings as soon as possible to disseminate current American information on the subject among surgeons across the country.

Slide 31   Listening to Saklad's lectures, Maeda was aware that Japan was far behind the United States in the specialty. The following year, in 1951, Maeda delivered a presidential lecture, entitled "We are in dire need of education and research in anesthesiology." at the 51st Annual Meeting of the JSS.[2] As shown in this slide, his lecture consisted of six topics, including a brief history of anesthesia in Japan, the education system in medical schools in the United States, and the education of anesthesia specialists. Maeda alluded to Saito's study of spinal anesthesia in the first topic because it was one of the most significant pieces of clinical research on anesthesia before 1950 in Japan. He concluded his lecture with the following sentence: "We have to urgently introduce American anesthesiology to our country and develop our own basic and clinical studies on the subject. I earnestly hope you will brace yourself up."

1. Maeda W. ed. *The Most Recent Surgery and Anesthesia*. Tokyo, Shindan to Chiryosha, 1951.
2. Maeda W. We are in dire need of education and research in anesthesiology. *J. Japan Surgical Society* 1952; 52: 566–8.

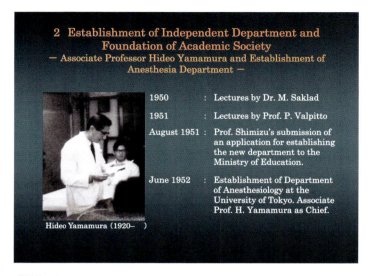

Slide 32

Slide 33

Slide 32   Some of the Japanese professors of surgery encouraged by Saklad and Maeda were exposed to Professor Volpitto's (1905–1988) lectures and demonstrations of clinical anesthesia in 1951.[1,2] He visited Japan as a member of the second medical mission. Among them, Kentaro Shimizu (1903–1987), a professor of the First Department of Surgery at the University of Tokyo, who studied at the University of Illinois both before and after the Pacific War and served as Saklad's translator, thought it essential to establish an independent department of anesthesiology for founding and developing the specialty.[3] He was also much concerned with neurosurgery, and realized that simultaneous progress in these two specialties was essential. Consequently, the first independent department of anesthesiology was established at the University of Tokyo in July 1952, and Hideo Yamamura (1920–), lecturer and chief of the anesthesia division under Shimizu, was appointed associate professor and chief of the newly established department.[4] The left–hand side of the slide shows Yamamura reading his paper in Shimizu's department.

Slide 33   Much attention should be paid to the relationship between the years in which the first independent departments of anesthesia were established and anesthesia societies were founded in Japan and abroad. As illustrated in this slide, the JSA was founded in 1954, 2 years after the establishment of the first independent department of anesthesia in 1952; in contrast, anesthesia societies in other countries were founded earlier than their corresponding departments.[5] This meant that no Japanese physician was specialized in anesthesia before 1950, and there was no basis for forming a meeting or society devoted to the subject. Therefore, there was a fundamental difference in the process of departmental establishment and foundation of societies between Japan and other countries.

1. Matsuki A. *The Origin of Anesthesiology, continued.* p.102–20.
2. Matsuki A. *A Short History of Anesthesia in Japan.* p.166–9.
3. ibid. p.169–73.
4. ibid. p.171.
5. ibid. p.177–8.

Increased Anesthesia-related Papers in JSS and JAFTS

Year	JSS Total Free Papers	JSS Anesthesia-related Papers (%)	JAFTS Total Free Papers	JAFTS Anesthesia-related Papers (%)
1949	60	0 (0)	76	0 (0)
1950	56	2 (3.6)	44	0 (0)
1951	113	7 (6.2)	111	8 (7.2)
1952	61	6 (9.8)	142	13 (9.2)
1953	84	2 (2.4)	170	16 (9.4)
1954	133	12 (9.0)	183	0 (0)
1955	134	0 (0)	166	1 (0.6)

Slide 34

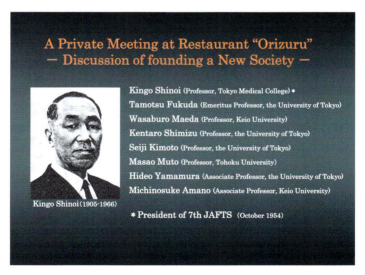

Slide 35

Slide 34   Within several years of the lectures by Saklad, Volpitto, and Maeda, "anesthesia" became the most important topic of study in surgical departments across the country. This slide shows the number of anesthesia–related presentations at the annual meetings of the JSS and Japanese Association for Thoracic Surgery (JAFTS) in the period 1949–1955. At both meetings, the number of anesthesia–related papers markedly increased after 1951, supporting the dominant influence of Saklad's lecture. The increased number of papers resulted in a tight schedule at the meetings, particularly at the JAFTS meeting. Professor Kingo Shinoi of the Tokyo Medical College, Tokyo, was the president of the Seventh Annual Meeting of the JAFTS to be held in October 1954. He expected that he would have a difficulty in arranging the anesthesia–related presentations in the program, and he came to the conclusion that there would be no alternative to founding a new society, at which anesthesia–related papers would be exclusively read.

Slide 35   As shown in this slide, Shinoi and several eminent professors of the JAFTS in the Tokyo area, Yamamura, and Michinosuke Amano, a lecturer at the Division of Anesthesia at Keio University, held a meeting in January 1954 to discuss the possibility of founding a new society in which only anesthesia–related papers would be presented, thereby avoiding a tight schedule at the Seventh JAFTS meeting. They arrived at the unanimous conclusion that a new society should be founded as early as possible. The delegate members at the meeting of the JSS in May 1954 formally approved the plan.[1] Subsequently, the JSA (its former appellation was the Japan Society of Anesthesiology) was practically separated from the JAFTS and formally divided from the JSS.

1. Anonym. The Japan Society of Anesthesiology established. *J. Japan Surgical Society* 2000; 101 (Supplement): 211.

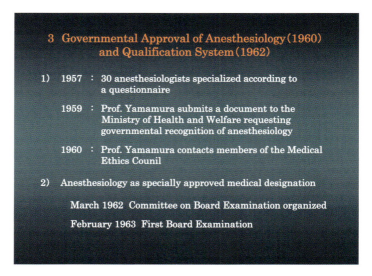

Slide 36

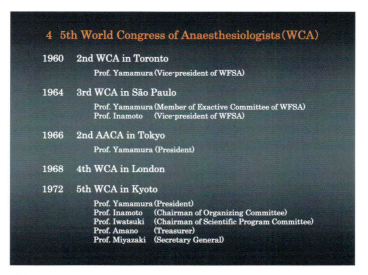

Slide 37

Slide 36   Although the JSA was founded in 1954 and anesthesia departments were gradually established in several schools of medicine in the 1950s, "anesthesia" was still unfamiliar as a discipline of clinical science among physicians and lay people. This is proven by the fact that only 30 physicians were specialized in anesthesia in 1957. As shown in this slide, Yamamura and some executive members of the society, together with members of the Tokyo Society of Anesthesiologists, endeavored to meet the following personnel to petition for the approval of anesthesiology as a designated specialty: Hiroshige Shiota (1873–1965), president of the Medical Ethics Committee of the Ministry of Health and Welfare; Taro Takemi (1904–1983), president of the Japan Medical Association; and officials of the Ministry of Health and Welfare. Finally, the petition was accepted in 1960, and the society established a system to qualify board certified anesthesiologists in 1962. Thus, the society launched the first qualification system in medical practice in Japan. This is one of the most significant events in the history of our specialty after 1950.[1-3]

Slide 37   Although the society was founded and the qualification system developed, it was necessary to hold a large international congress to exchange information on the specialty with foreign researchers and clinicians and prove Japanese standards of the specialty to meet international standards. In 1964, at the third WCA in São Paulo, Yamamura was approached by some influential members of the congress about hosting the fourth WCA in 1968; however, he declined the proposal because the JSA was not ready to hold an international meeting. Two years later, in 1966, the second Asian Australasian Congress of Anaesthesiologists was held in Tokyo under the presidency of Yamamura. The JSA's well-organized management impressed eminent members from other countries. This success led to Japan being nominated as the host country for the fifth WCA in 1972 by an Executive Committee meeting and its unanimous approval at the general assembly at the fourth WCA held in London in 1968.

1. Yamamura H. Historical Details on the Emergence of Registered Anesthesiologists and Board Certified Anesthesiologists in Japan. In Fujita T. and Matsuki A. eds. *The History of Japanese Anesthesiology. Source Materials.* (Vol.1) Tokyo, Kokuseido Shuppan, 1987. p.63–8.
2. Matsuki A. *A Short History of Anesthesia in Japan.* p.189–92.
3. Matsuki A. The Background for Governmental Accreditation of "Anesthesiology" as a Specially Approved Medical Specialty. (1) and (2). *Masui* 2014; 63: 594–9, 706–11.

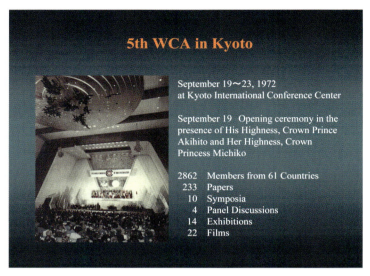

Slide 38

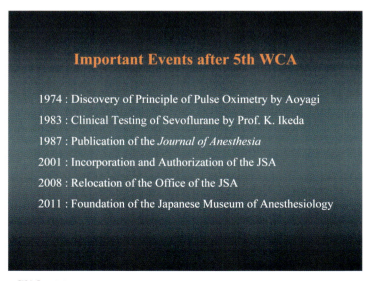

Slide 39

Slide 38   The fifth WCA was held in Kyoto from September 19–23, 1972. The left–hand side of the slide shows the opening ceremony of the congress. On September 19, the opening ceremony was conducted in the presence of His Highness, Crown Prince Akihito, and Her Highness, Crown Princess Michiko [presently, His Majesty (the Emperor) and Her Majesty (the Empress)] . In total, 2862 members from 61 countries participated in the congress, at which 233 papers were presented; 10 symposia, four panel discussions, 14 scientific exhibitions were held; and 22 films were screened.[1–3]

Slide 39   This slide illustrates several significant discoveries in anesthesia and activities of the society in Japan after the fifth WCA. The foundation of associated academic and subspecialty societies, together with significant research conducted in many institutions, should be mentioned in this lecture; however, I am forced to abbreviate them because of time constraints.

1. Inamoto A. A reminiscence of the 5th World Congress of Anaesthesiologists. *Rinsho Masui* 1973; 2: 357–63.
2. Iwatsuki K. A report from the Academic Program Committee of the 5th World Congress of Anaesthesiologists. *Masui* 1973; 22: 101–5.
3. Matsuki A. *A Short History of Anesthesia in Japan.* p.202–3.

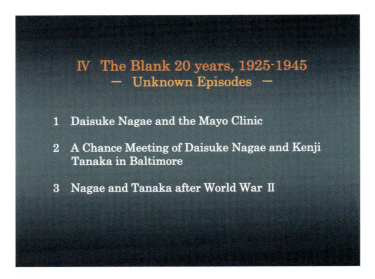

Slide 40

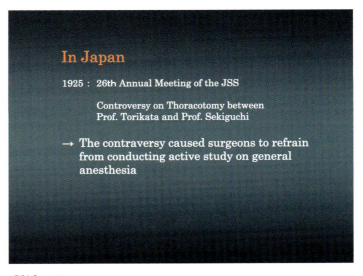

Slide 41

4   The Blank 20 Years, 1925–1945

Slide 40   I have briefly described the 60-year-history of anesthesia in Japan since 1950. Reflecting on our history between 1868 (the Meiji Restoration) and the very early years of the 21st century, it is apparent that the advancement of anesthesiology in Japan was hampered before the outbreak of the Pacific War in the 1920s and 1930s. I will now discuss these hindrances further in the fourth chapter, entitled "The Blank 20 Years, 1925–1945," and explain them in three sections.

Slide 41   Since the middle of the Meiji era, Japanese surgeons had attached more importance to the use of local anesthesia than to that of general anesthesia during surgery, and this tradition had been uninterruptedly passed down until the end of the Pacific War.

According to previous studies on the history of our specialty, a surgical controversy was thought to underlie the hindrance of the advancement of anesthesia. In 1925, a controversy arose at the 26th Annual Meeting of the JSS between Ryuzo Torikata (1878–1952), professor of surgery at Kyoto University, Kyoto, Japan, and Shigeki Sekiguchi (1880–1942), professor of surgery at Tohoku University, Sendai, Japan, on the optimum method of thoracotomy. Torikata insisted that thoracotomy could and should be performed without assisted positive–pressure ventilation and that positive–pressure ventilation was a contraindication with grave surgical outcomes. Sekiguchi objected, insisting on its efficacy. The debate between them was so fierce that the audience in the hall fell silent. The controversy lasted for the subsequent 10 years.

Unfortunately, because Torikata was one of the most eminent and influential professors in the JSS at that time, his views caused surgeons to refrain from conducting active research on general anesthesia and positive–pressure ventilation during anesthesia.[1]

---

1. Inamoto A. Learning from the History of a Medical Controversy in Japan–in relation to thoracotomy with no positive–pressure ventilation–. *Japanese J. Clinical Anesthesia* 1994; 14: 36–8.

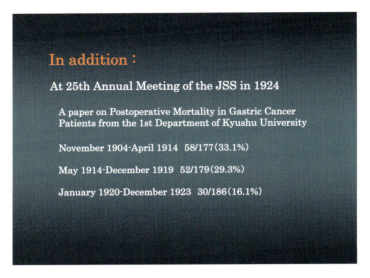

Slide 42

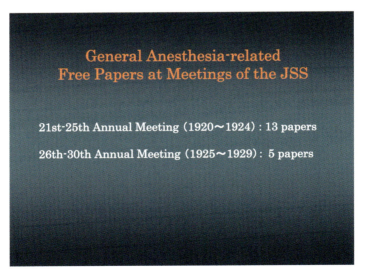

Slide 43

Slide 42 In 1924, just 1 year before the start of the controversy, an attractive paper[1] was presented at the 25th Annual Meeting of the JSS by Professor Miyake's (1867–1945) Department of Surgery at Kyushu University, Fukuoka, Japan. As shown in this slide, they reported that the postoperative mortality rates of patients with gastric cancer (within 1 month of surgery) were 33.1% in the period November 1904–April 1914, and 29.3% in the period May 1914–December 1919. Chloroform was used as the main general anesthetic agent during these two periods. Miyake surmised that chloroform itself may have a deleterious effect on postoperative outcomes and decided to use local anesthesia instead of chloroform anesthesia. This resulted in a dramatic improvement in postoperative mortality rates. The mortality rate for the next 4 years between January 1920–December 1923 was 16.3%, almost a half of that in the preceding two periods.[2] This paper must have been responsible for a negative impact on surgeons, discouraging them from using general anesthesia and positive pressure ventilation.

Slide 43 These two factors had a serious impact on surgeons across the country. This is proven by the numbers of anesthesia–related papers at the annual meetings of the JSS before1924 and after 1925, when the paper from Miyake's department was presented. As shown in this slide, anesthesia–related papers presented during 5 years between 1920–1924 totaled 13, whereas they markedly deceased to 5 (40% of 13) in the next 5 years between 1925 and 1929. These data suggest that Japanese surgeons at that time were not strongly concerned about general anesthesia, anesthetics, and the practice of anesthesia. This is the reason why I entitled this section "The Blank 20 Years, 1925–1945."[2,3]

1. Taniguchi K. Postoperative Results of Gastric Cancer Patients of the First Department of Surgery, Kyushu University. *J. Japan Surgical Society*. 1924; 25: 1418–87.
2. Professor Miyake described the detailed results of surgical operations on gastric patients in the following monograph.
   Miyake H, Miyagi J, and Taniguchi K. *Gastric Cancer*. Tokyo, Kokuseido Shuppan, 1928.
3. This issue is discussed in the Section 4 of the Chapter Ⅲ.

Chapter I　The Origin and Evolution of Anesthesia in Japan

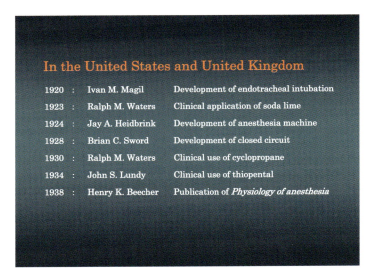

Slide 44

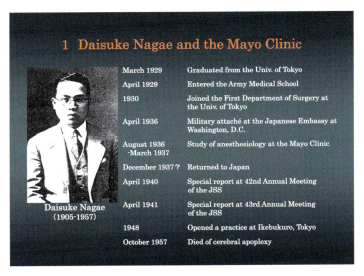

Slide 45

Slide 44   In the 1920s and 1930s, remarkable advances were made in the field of anesthesia in the United States and United Kingdom. As shown in this slide, effective general anesthetics and useful anesthetic methods were developed, and new anesthetic machines and a closed–circuit system were devised, most of which form the basis of modern anesthesiology.[1-3] Unfortunately, Japanese surgeons ignored the advances in both countries.

Slide 45   There is a proverb "There is no rule without exceptions," and one exception was Daisuke Nagae (1905–1957),[4] who understood the importance and significance of anesthesia in the surgical care of patients and advocated modern American anesthesiology. As illustrated in this slide, he graduated from the University of Tokyo. Subsequently, he entered the Army Medical School for financial reasons, and graduated in 1930. He joined the First Department of Surgery at the University of Tokyo, presided over by Professor Tetsuzo Aoyama (1882–1953), as a research fellow and studied surgery. He obtained a Ph.D. and became an instructor in the Division of Surgery at the Army Medical School in 1936. Soon after that, the Army Medical School requested that Nagae go abroad to study in the United States. He worked as a military attaché at the Japanese Embassy in Washington, D.C. His daily activities in the United States are unknown; however, it is noteworthy that he remained at the Mayo Clinic, Rochester, Minnesota, as a volunteer research fellow for 8 months and studied anesthesia under John S. Lundy (1893–1973). He returned to Japan in December 1937. After his return, he worked for the Army Medical School teaching thoracic surgery, and presented his papers at the 42nd and 43rd Annual Meetings of the JSS in 1941 and 1942. After the end of the Pacific War, he opened a practice at Ikebukuro, Tokyo, in 1948. He died of cerebral apoplexy in 1957. He was the only Japanese to study anesthesia in a foreign country for more than 6 months before 1945.

1. Keys TE. *The History of Surgical Anesthesia*. New York, Schuman's, 1945.
2. Rushman GB, Davies NJH, and Atkinson RS. *A Short History of Anaesthesia. The first 150 Years*. 1996.
3. Volpitto PP, and Vandam L. eds. *The Genesis of Contemporary Anesthesiology*. Springfield, CC Thomas, 1982.
4. Matsuki A. *A Short History of Anesthesia in Japan*. p.153–6.

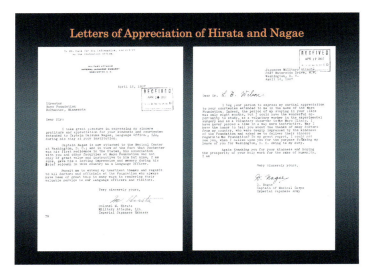

Slide 46

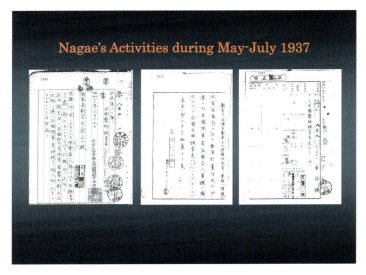

Slide 47

Slide 46   This slide shows documents provided by the Historical Unit of the Mayo Clinic. The left–hand side of the slide shows a letter of appreciation by Masachika Hirata (1891–1960), a colonel and Nagae's superior at the Japanese Embassy in Washington, D.C. The letter was addressed to the director of the Mayo Clinic to express his thanks for their kind arrangements for Nagae. The right–hand side of the slide depicts a letter written by Nagae to Dr. L.B. Wilson of the clinic, to whom Nagae was much obliged during his stay at the clinic.

Slide 47   Nagae's daily activities remain unclear after his return to Washington, D.C. from the Mayo Clinic, however, it is evident from Hirata's letter that Nagae was studying at the "Medical Center in Washington, D.C." Nagae had several chances to visit notable hospitals for the purpose of observing thoracic surgical operations. One of Nagae's duties as the military attaché was to collect information from American army surgeons. This slide shows a letter by Hirata addressed to the Ministry of War of Japan, relating that a sample of a "personal card" of a United Army physician was privately collected by Nagae.

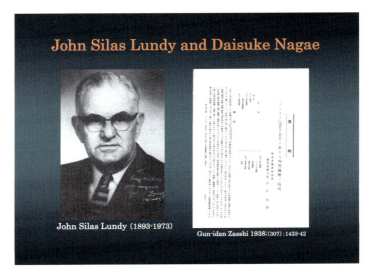

Slide 48

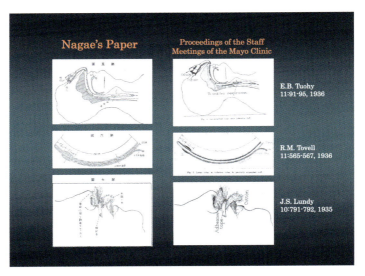

Slide 49

Slide 48   When Nagae stayed at the Mayo Clinic, John S. Lundy (1893–1973) was the chief of the Department of Anesthesia at the clinic. The left–hand side of the slide shows a photograph of Dr. Lundy. Nagae had a hard time studying anesthesiology, and after returning to Japan, he published a paper reporting his experiences at the clinic, which appeared in the *Gun–idan Zasshi* (*Army Surgeons' Journal*) in 1938,[1] as shown in the right–hand side of the slide. The paper is entitled "*Recent State of Surgical Anesthesia at the Mayo Clinic.*"

Slide 49   The left–hand side of the slide illustrates the figures that appeared in Nagae's paper, all taken from the journal *Proceedings of the Staff Meeting of the Mayo Clinic.*[2-4] Edward Boyce Tuohy (1908–1959), Ralph M. Tovell (1901–1967), and John S. Lundy were well– known anesthesiologists at the clinic.

1. Nagae D. Recent state of surgical anesthesia at the Mayo Clinic. *Gun–idan Zasshi* 1938; (307): 1433–42.
2. Tuohy EB. Intratracheal anesthesia. *Proceedings of the Staff Meeting of the Mayo Clinic*. 1936; 11: 91–5.
3. Tovell RM. A New Intratracheal tube. *Proceedings of the Staff Meeting of the Mayo Clinic*. 1936; 11: 565–7.
4. Lundy JS. A method of minimizing respiratory depression when using soluble barbiturates intravenously. *Proceedings of the Staff Meeting of the Mayo Clinic*. 1935; 10: 791–2.

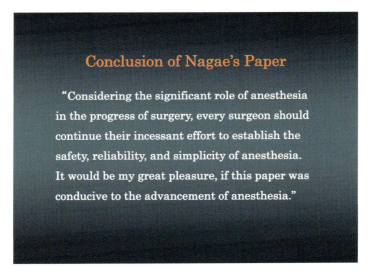

Slide 50

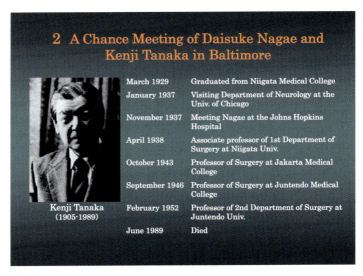

Slide 51

Slide 50   Nagae concluded his paper as shown in the slide.

> Considering the significant role of anesthesia in the progress of surgery, every surgeon should continue their incessant effort to establish the safety, reliability, and simplicity of anesthesia. It would be my great pleasure if this paper was conducive to the advancement of anesthesia.[1]

I have no hesitation in terming him one of the pioneers of modern anesthesiology in Japan, because he had a deeper insight and more definite perspective of modern American anesthesiology than any other Japanese surgeon at the time.

Slide 51   Even after completing his study at the Mayo Clinic, Nagae continued studying surgery despite a hectic workload and attempted to make visits to several hospitals. In November 1937, he visited Johns Hopkins University Hospital at Baltimore for the purpose of observing a thoracotomy performed by Associate Professor William F. Rienhoff, Jr. (1894–1981). In the operating theater at the hospital, Nagae happened to come across Kenji Tanaka (1905–1989), a Japanese surgeon from Niigata University, Niigata, Japan, who was visiting the hospital to observe Professor Walter Dandy's (1886–1946) neurosurgical procedures. He was a research fellow at Percival Bailey's Department of Neurosurgery at the University of Chicago.[2] The slide contains a photograph and short biography of Tanaka. It was a great coincidence that Nagae met Tanaka in the operating theater, where they realized that both Japanese thoracic surgery and neurosurgery were lagging far behind the United States and concluded that the study of anesthesiology, particularly tracheal anesthesia, would be indispensable for achieving rapid improvement in these two specialties in Japan. Tanaka wrote a paper on modern American anesthesia during his stay in Baltimore, which appeared in the Japanese journal *Geka*.[3]

1. Nagae D. Recent state of surgical anesthesia at the Mayo Clinic. *Gun–idan Zasshi* 1938; (307): 1442.
2. Matsuki A. *Japanese Pioneers in Anesthesiology– An Introduction to the Study of the History of Anesthesiology.* Tokyo, Kokuseido Shuppan, 1983. p.74–81.
3. Tanaka K. The second step in neurosurgery. *Geka* 1938; 2: 1161–71.

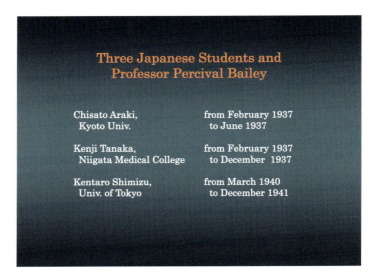

Slide 52

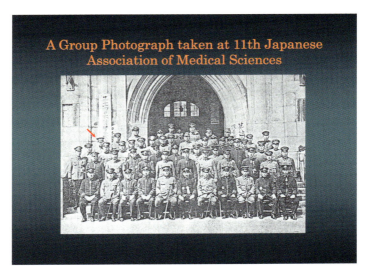

Slide 53

Slide 52 I would like to introduce to you one more important person Chisato Araki (1901–1976), a surgeon from Kyoto University and a disciple of Torikata. He was also a research fellow at Professor Percival Bailey's (1892–1973) Department at the University of Chicago. Thus, Araki and Tanaka were studying in the same department. Araki had many concerns about anesthesiology and neurosurgery. As shown in this slide, Bailey's department was deeply connected with Japanese surgeons because these three surgeons studied under him in the 1930s and 1940s, and they would go on to play important roles in anesthesia in the 1950s in Japan. Araki[1-4] wrote several papers on American neurosurgery that appeared in the Journal *Geka Hokan* edited by Torikata; however, in them, the anesthetic management of neurosurgical patients was described in least detail. This is most likely because of Araki's intention to avoid making an unfavorable impression on Torikata. In 1956, Akira Inamoto (1909–2001), a junior colleague of Araki, became the first professor of Anesthesiology at Kyoto University, the fourth independent department in Japan.

Slide 53 Tanaka remembered clearly that he met Nagae at the Annual Meetings of the JSS in 1941 and 1942, where they discussed the importance of tracheal anesthesia; however, most senior surgeons of the JSS did not. This slide illustrates a group photograph taken at the joint session of the JSS and the Military Medical Association at the 11th Japanese Association of Medical Sciences Meeting in 1942. Mrs. Tami Tohyama (1929–), the eldest daughter of Nagae, identified her father (red arrow) in the photograph.

1. Araki C. A report from instructor Araki in the United States. *Geka Hokan* 1936; 13: 819–31.
2. Araki C. A perspctive of Professor Dandy's neurosurgery. *Geka Hokan* 1937; 14: 241–72.
3. Araki C. A report of visits to the neurosurgical departments in Philadelphia and New Haven. *Geka Hokan* 1937; 14: 590–616.
4. Araki C. Neurosurgical studies by Professor Dandy. *Geka Hokan* 1937; 14: 799–825.

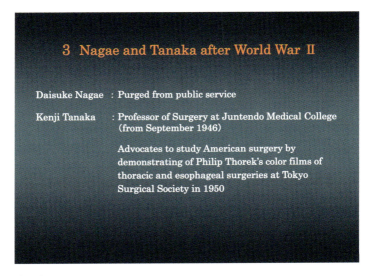

Slide 54

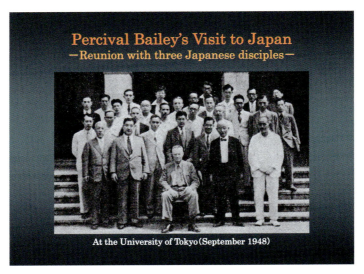

Slide 55

Slide 54   After the end of the Pacific War, Nagae was one of many people purged from public service between 1946 and 1951 because he had been colonel army surgeon. Subsequently, he opened a surgical practice at Ikebukuro, Tokyo in 1948. Tanaka became a professor of surgery at Juntendo Medical College, Tokyo, where he strived to introduce American surgery. He became acquainted with Dr. S.E. Moolten(?–?), a major of the GHQ responsible for the introduction of internships in Japan, and borrowed from him color films featuring Philip Thorek's surgical operations to demonstrate at the 492nd Meeting of the Tokyo Surgical Society in November 1950 in Tokyo.[1] The films created a fresh and vivid impression on every surgeon in attendance, because the surgical procedures of the thorax and esophagus they demonstrated had been performed without exception under tracheal anesthesia. Tanaka also made every effort to encourage young physicians and medical students to study in the United States.

Slide 55   On August 24, 1948, Kentaro Shimizu, Associate professor at the First Department of Surgery at the University of Tokyo, received an unexpected telephone call from GHQ asking him to come to the Imperial Hotel at five o'clock in the afternoon to see Professor Bailey, his previous mentor at the University of Illinois.[2] Although Bailey visited Japan at the request of GHQ and not the Japanese government, the true purpose of his visit to Japan remains unclear. Shimizu took the rare opportunity to ask Bailey to give a lecture on neurology. Bailey accepted Shimizu's proposal and the lecture, entitled "Recent Developments in Neurology,"[3] was delivered on September 1 at the University of Tokyo. Shimizu was the translator at the lecture. This slide shows a group photograph taken just after the lecture.[4] A number of eminent professors who played important roles in establishing the departments of anesthesia and founding the society can be seen in this photograph. Front row, left to right: Wasaburo Maeda of Keio University; Makoto Saito of Nagoya University; Professor Bailey; and Takeo Tamiya, the Dean of the Faculty of Medicine at the University of Tokyo. Kenji Tanaka is behind Professor Bailey; Kentaro Shimizu is on Tanaka's left; and Chisato Araki is on the right of Tanaka. On this occasion, Maeda realized Shimizu's proficiency in English; Shimizu would go on to act as an interpreter for Saklad 2 years later.

1. Kuwabara S. A Dialogue of A and B who attended at the 492nd Meeting of the Tokyo Surgical Society. *Geka* 1950; 12: 717–21.
2. Shimizu K. Postscript. *Brain and Nerves*. 1949; (5): 346.
3. Bailey P. Recent Developments in Neurology. *Brain and Nerves*. 1949; (2): 78–91.
4. The photograph appeared in the Vol.1 No.1 issue of *Brain and Nerves* in 1948.

V Historical Perspective

1. International Exchange
2. Social Status of Anesthesiologists
3. Preservation of Historic Documents

Slide 56

1 International Exchange

1. North America : U.S. and Canada
2. Europe : U.K., Germany, France, and Scandinavia
3. Asia : China, Korea
4. Oceania : Australia and New Zealand

Slide 57

5 From Historical Perspective

Slide 56   Finally, I have come to the last chapter of my lecture. This slide shows the contents of this chapter. It consists of the following three sections:

1. uninterrupted international exchange with foreign countries;
2. improvement in the social status of anesthesiologists and the specialty of anesthesiology; and
3. preservation of historical documents and compilation of a database on the history of the specialty.

Slide 57   It is mandatory for us to have friendly and uninterrupted exchange with colleagues in the countries shown in this slide. At present, the relationship between Japan and the United States is too close, which is frankly reminiscent of the situation of a few decades before the Pacific War, when we exchanged information with Germany alone and ignored the United States and United Kingdom. These circumstances should be improved as soon as possible. I hear that the executive members of the JSA have been working hard on this issue. We Japanese tend to pay more attention to technical facets of things than to their backgrounds. Ken–ichi Iwatsuki (1913–2013), an emeritus professor of Tohoku University, Sendai, Japan, expressed the view that adopting a technique alone from another country is like aimlessly drifting with the current, and does not represent an advance of significance. We must keep his words firmly in mind.[1]

1. Iwatsuki K. The reasons that I became an anesthesiologist. *Anet* 1988; 2: 21–2.

Chapter I The Origin and Evolution of Anesthesia in Japan

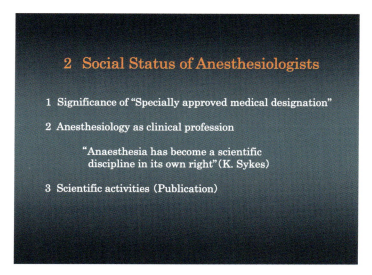

Slide 58

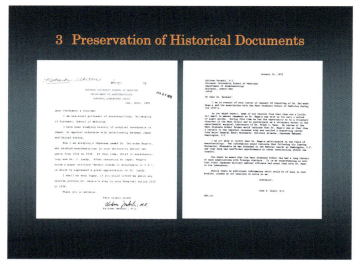

Slide 59

Slide 58   It is necessary for us to consider the social status of anesthesiologists and the social position of our society. Therefore, we must pay deliberate attention to our "specially approved designation," which differs from "generally approved designations" such as internal medicine, surgery, orthopedics, and gynecology. Although the Ministry of Health, Labor, and Welfare revised the designation system in 2008, our "specially approved designation" remains unchanged. One possible solution for this issue is that the society has just revised the qualification system for "board certified anesthesiologists."

Our society includes a large number of members, almost all of whom are anesthesiologists. The Emeritus Professor Michinosuke Amano (1916–), one of the founders of the society, repeatedly emphasized that each of us should be seriously aware of being an anesthesiologist.[1,2] According to our history, neither the first independent department of anesthesiology nor the society was founded by anesthesiologists. Amano's words remind us that we must be more conscious of ourselves as anesthesiologists. A similar edifying intention has been repeatedly expressed by the Emeritus Professor Hisayo O. Morishima (1929–) of Columbia University, New York City, on many occasions.

According to Professor Kazuyoshi Hirota (1959–) of Hirosaki University, Hirosaki, Japan, the Editor-in-Chief of the *Journal of Anesthesia*, the publication of papers by Japanese researchers in major English journals related to the specialty has decreased in recent years. The social status of our society largely rests on our academic activities, therefore, it is strongly necessary that this situation improves rapidly.

Slide 59   In the third section, I am going to talk about the preservation of historical documents and compilation of a database on the history of our specialty. Last year, I sent an e-mail to the Mayo Clinic requesting further information on Nagae. They kindly supplied me with some important documents on him together with my letter addressed to the clinic in 1978, as shown in the left-hand side of the slide. This indicates that the clinic has an excellent database, and they can supply us with data by e-mail within hours. Considering this situation, we must admit that the tremendous gap in the specialty in the 1950s between Japan and the United States is reflected in the compilation of this database in the 2010s. Using our immature database system, it will be arduous to undertake historical studies on the specialty; however, they should be considered mandatory for raising our social status.

1. Amano M. Philosophy of anesthesiology. *Respiration and Circulation* 1961; 9: 607.
2. Private communication with Professor Amano in 1987.

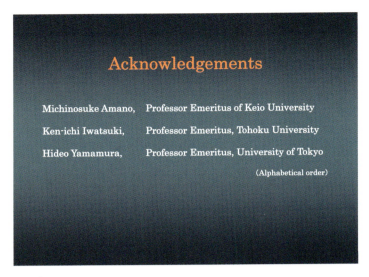

Slide 60

Slide 60   This is the final slide of my lecture. I would like to extend my cordial thanks to the many senior members of the society who have helped me by providing a lot of precious advice. If you find anything significant in my lecture, it must be suggestions from these three great pioneers: Michinosuke Amano, Ken–ichi Iwatsuki,[1] and Hideo Yamamura (alphabetical order), who gave me invaluable lessons. For this, I have to express my profound appreciation to these pioneers of the society. Once again, I wish to express my profound gratitude to Professor Iwasaki for inviting me to participate in this meeting. Thank you very much for your careful attention.

1. Professor Ken–ichi Iwatsuki passed away on November 20, 2013.

Chapter II History of Anesthesia in Japan before 1867

Five topics related to the history of anesthesia in Japan before 1867 are discussed in this chapter. Readers may notice an inconsistency between this chapter featuring 1867 as a period division and the previous book, *A Short History of Anesthesia in Japan* (2012), featuring 1804, 1850, and 1898 as division periods. The previous division periods in the book are useful for understanding and discussing the history of anesthesiology in Japan within the context of anesthesia and medical sciences in general. However, the year 1868 has an important significance in the history in Japan that should not be neglected when discussing the history of medicine associated with the adoption of the German style of medicine by the Meiji Government (1868–1912). A significant theme in this book is the retardation of advancements in anesthesiology in the 1920s and 1930s, and one of the causative factors for this impediment is considered the adoption of the German style of medicine in the very early years of the Meiji era. Consequently, I considered pre–1867 and post–1868 as distinct eras.

1   Tokumei Takamine Did not Administer General Anesthetics in Ryukyu

The prevailing opinion among medical historians half a century ago in Japan was that Tokumei Takamine (1653–1738, Chinese name, Wei Shizhe; Japanese pronunciation, Gi Shitetsu), a bureaucrat of the Ryukyu Kingdom (presently Okinawa), may have administered general anesthetics more than 100 years before Seishu Hanaoka (1760–1835). This belief originated from Kanjun Higashionna (1882–1963), a native historian of Okinawa, who wrote an essay on the medical history of Okinawa in 1954, which appeared in a local newspaper, *Ryukyu Shimpo*.[1] He mentioned in the essay that Takamine may have performed cleft lip surgery using a general anesthetic called "Mafutsusan." He repeated this view in another historical essay on medicine in Okinawa in the same newspaper the following year.[2] His conviction of Takamine's administration of general anesthesia was summarized in an article published in 1958.[3]

However, Higashionna's insistence on the subject was a result of his

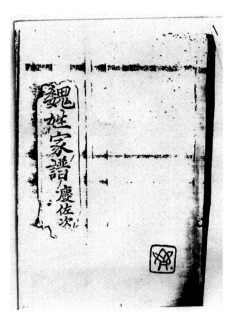

Figure 2.1.1 Title page of the "*Gisei Kafu*."

misinterpretation of the Gi Family's Genealogy (*Gisei Kafu* in Chinese, Figure 2.1.1) because neither a description of Takamine's supposed practice of general anesthesia nor the word "Mafutsusan" is found in the genealogy, as shown later. The "*Gisei Kafu*" is the only extant historical document describing Takamine's life. This document makes it apparent that Higashionna misinterpreted the meaning of genealogy as if Takamine used general anesthetic "Mafutsusan" in cleft lip operations. However, this erroneous account was widely disseminated in Japan when Kiyomatsu Kinjo (1880–1974), a physician and medical historian from Okinawa, read a paper in 1963 on the medical history of Okinawa, including Higashionna's view on Takamine, before the 64th Annual Meeting of the Japanese Society of Medical History.[4] In 1976, Kinjo published *A Chronology of Medicine in Ryukyu*,[5] wherein he described Takamine's use of general anesthesia. Because this has been the only authoritative textbook on the medical history of Okinawa, Higashionna's misconception was firmly established across Japan. Considering that a recent publication of Takamine's biography prominently features his use of general anesthesia,[6] this deceptive information continues to influence medical historians in Japan.

It is necessary to appreciate the background of Takamine's life before discussing Higashionna's opinion. At the time of Takamine, the Ryukyu Islands were ruled by King Shotei (1645–1709), the 11th King of the Ryukyu Kingdom (the Second Sho Dynasty, 1469–1879). Unfortunately, his grandson Shoeki (the 12th King, 1678–1712) had a cleft lip. The King was seriously concerned about his grandson's deformity, as Shoeki was to succeed to the throne. In 1688, Takamine visited Fuzhou, China, as a member of the official mission of the Kingdom to China because he was proficient in Chinese. Sen–yu Omine, one of the superior members of the mission, happened to hear that Huang Hui–you, an itinerant Chinese physician, was in Nantai near Fuzhou, China, to repair a cleft lip. His brother–in–law Yonamine, a captain of the ships of the mission, was suffering from a cleft lip, so Omine and Yonamine visited Huang and entreated him to repair Yonamine's defect, a surgery that was eventually performed successfully. Observing this success, the other superior members of the mission, who had been anxious about Shoeki's deformity, ordered Takamine to acquire the technique of cleft lip surgery from Huang since Takamine had the best command of Chinese among the delegates. He was initially reluctant to accept their request because he was not a physician, however, they persuaded him by repeatedly emphasizing that to master the technique would be an enormous contribution to both the happiness of the royal family and the future prosperity of the Kingdom.

Despite the earnest and repeated pleadings of Takamine, Huang obstinately refused to disclose or teach him the surgical technique because it was a family secret handed down from parent to child. Takamine appealed to him for several days by explaining that the royal family of the Kingdom was in a serious predicament and that disclosing the technique to him would be an exceptional case because he was a foreigner. At last, Huang submitted to his urgent plea and introduced him to the technique, which Takamine avidly practiced for 20 days. His training was completed in February 1689 when he successfully repaired a 13–year–old patient's cleft lip in the presence of Huang, after which Huan gave Takamine a scroll describing the secrets of the procedure.

Takamine returned to Ryukyu together with the other members of the mission in May 1689. The King and Prince Shojun (1660–1707), Shoeki's father, were delighted to hear that Takamine had mastered the skill of repairing a cleft lip from Huang Hui–you. In an attempt to assure the safety of the procedure, they ordered Takamine to examine whether a concoction of indigenous ingredients would have the same effects as the Chinese mixture used by Huang. In addition, to confirm his skill, they asked him to conduct

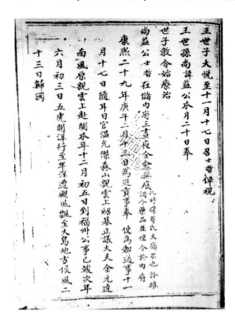

Figure 2.1.2　Account of November and December 1689 in "*Gisei Kafu.*" The first four lines are translated into English.

preliminary surgeries on several patients, and Takamine successfully treated five cleft lip patients within approximately 3 months after August 1689. Once assured of his skill, Shojun permitted him to proceed, and he succeeded in treating Shoeki's cleft lip on November 20, 1689.

At that time, the Ryukyu Kingdom was under the control of the Shimazu or Satsuma Domain (presently Kagoshima Prefecture), which accredited a magistrate to the Kingdom. In September 1690, at the request of Genzaemon Murao (?–?), a magistrate of Ryukyu dispatched by the Shimazu Domain, Takamine demonstrated a cleft lip surgery to Doyo Isashiki (1661–1730), a feudal physician from the Shimazu Domain, and gave him a scroll describing the secrets of the surgery. Takamine donated another copy of the scroll to Murao.

Takamine's cleft lip surgery on Shoeki is described in an account of the "*Gisei Kafu*" from November and December 1689 (Figure 2.1.2). It reads as follows:

> The Prince (Shojun) was absolutely delighted (to have observed Takamine's successful preliminary surgeries on five patients) and ordered Shitetsu (Takamine's other given name) to proceed to the court and examine Shoeki, which he did on November 17 (1689).

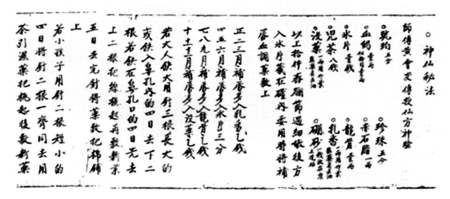

Figure 2.1.3 First part of the "*Shinsen Hiho*".

On November 20, Shitetsu began treating Shoeki by the order of the Prince Shojun at the court. Shitetsu stayed there for 3 days and nights, and Shoeki's defect was completely obliterated with no visible trace.

On this occasion, Takamine brought Sen-yu Omine with him to the court and asked him to concoct the drug and keep contact with the courtiers

(Words in parentheses are supplementary annotations by the author.)

It is evident that neither the term "general anesthesia" nor the term "Mafutsusan" is found in these accounts from the "*Gisei Kafu*," and there is not even an allusion to "general anesthesia." In addition, these two terms are not found in a 1690 account of the cleft lip surgery in the genealogy. These facts strongly suggest that Takamine did not use general anesthetics. Consequently, it appears (although there is no definitive proof) that Higashionna misunderstood the nature of "the drug" described in the "*Gisei Kafu*." This issue will be discussed later.

I have attempted to investigate the lives of Isashiki and Murao, the recipients of the secret scrolls, and other facts related to Takamine's practice of cleft lip surgery. Dr. Yasumasa Isashiki (1921–2004), a direct descendant of Doyo Isashiki, was running a private ophthalmology practice in Kagoshima when I met him in 1977 to discuss Doyo Isashiki. He discovered that neither the scroll nor any related historical documents had been handed down in the family. Similarly, no information was obtained about the descendants of Murao or the fate of the scroll given to him. Since 1981, I have also visited Okinawa several times but have found no new information related to Takamine.

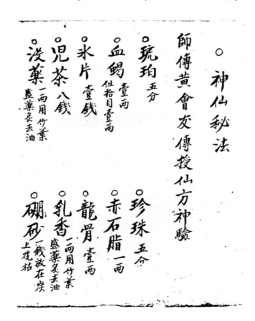

Figure 2.1.4 Formulae and Dispensing.

　　I surmised through repeated field surveys in Kagoshima and Okinawa that the two scrolls that Takamine had contributed to Isashiki and Murao or their copies are likely to be extant somewhere in Kagoshima Prefecture because people are apt to preserve such precious scrolls and asked colleagues and librarians in the area to search for them.

　　Fortunately, a copy of the scroll (Figure 2.1.3) was found in 1986 at Sendai, Kagoshima Prefecture.[7] This copy was donated by a direct descendent of a Shimazu feudal physician to the Sendai Historical Museum. The clarified provenance of the copy proves its reliability. The copy is entitled "*Shinsen Hiho*" (A Taoistic Secret) and measures 18 cm in width and 275 cm in length. It was transcribed in 1749 by Antei Kore-eda and Encho Nagai, who were likely feudal physicians of the Shimazu Domain; however, their biographies remain unknown.

　　The scroll contains the following descriptions: A Taoistic Secret (title), Miraculous Secret initiated by Huang Hui-you (subtitle), Formulae and Dispensing, Operative Method, Derivation of the Secret and its Initiation to Takamine, Signatures of Antei Kore-eda and Encho Nagai, Remarks on the Eldest Son of Hisayuki Shimazu[8] (a branch of the Shimazu feudal clan), and Several Miscellaneous Writings. The most important section is the Formulae and Dispensing (Figure 2.1.4). It reads as follows:

Amber, Pearl, Sanguinis draconis, Halloysite, Borneo camphor, Long-gu,* Gambier, Frankincense, Myrrh, and Borax.

After the midst of spring, 10 above-mentioned ingredients are to be ground and percolated. Then add Borneo camphor. Preserve in a container. When in use, mix with blood and apply it on the incision.

Increase dose of Frankincense for the operation in January, February, and March.
Increase dose of Borneo camphor for the operation in April, May, and June.
Increase dose of Long-gu* for the operation in July, August, and September.
Increase dose of Myrrh for the operation in October, November, and December.

(*Ryukotsu, fossils of ancient mammals,) (Unit abbreviated)

According to this description, the drug consists of 10 ingredients, none of which has anesthetic properties or potent analgesic effects. Each ingredient had been used as a component of ointments for traumatic and incisional wounds in the practice of traditional Chinese medicine, and the phrase "apply it on the incision" clearly indicates that the drug was an ointment. Consequently, it is apparent that the drug formula Takamine obtained from Huang was not for a general anesthetic but an ointment. Since the prescription is described first in the scroll, it was likely considered the most important aspect of the initiation.

Despite the 1986 discovery of "A Taoistic Secret" at Sendai, Kagoshima Prefecture, the erroneous opinion of Higashionna was still widely accepted. In 1995, a Committee was formed in Okinawa to investigate the activities of Huang Hui-you and Takamine in the Fuzhou area. Some of the committee members have made repeated visits to the area but have found no definitive proof of Huang's practice of general anesthesia. Considering that he had not used general anesthesia for cleft lip surgery, as evidenced by the copied scroll, it is unlikely that Takamine ever used general anesthesia. In 2011, Ikeda[9] discussed the possible use of general anesthesia by Takamine and his indirect influence on Hanaoka; this theory was rejected.

Before the publication of Ikeda's article, I published a paper concluding that every article on Takamine after Higashionna's 1954 essay incorrectly claims that Takamine had practiced general anesthesia.[10] I also conducted a detailed review of the documents associated with Takamine to show that the "*Gisei Kafu*" is still the only extant document mentioning Takamine's surgical treatment of Shoeki.[11] These papers[10,11] were written in Japanese to correct this aspect of history; Takamine did not use general anesthesia and therefore made no significant contribution to the subsequent development of anesthesia in Japan. I had direct communication with Professor Emeritus

Ikeda to discuss the subject. He earnestly advised the writing of this English language article on Takamine's "drug."

References and Remarks

1. Higashionna K. *Complete Works of Kanjun Higashionna*. (Vol.9) Tokyo, Daiichi Shobo, 1980. p.103–6.
2. Reference 1. p.8.
3. Higashionna K. Tokumei Takamine – A Pioneer of General Anesthesia for Surgery in Ryukyu–. *Itan* (reissue series) 1958; (18): 1789–93.
4. Kinjo K. An Outline of the Medical History of Ryukyu. Itan (reissue series) 1963; (28): 2117–28.
5. Kinjo K. *A Chronology of Medicine in Ryukyu*. Naha, Wakanatsu, 1976. p.85.
6. Matsumoto J. *Tokumei Takamine – A Pioneer of General Anesthesia*. Naha, Ryukyu Shimpo, 2007.
7. Ogura K. A Secret Scroll of Cleft Lip Surgery Bequeathed in the Satsuma Feudal Domain. *Sendai* 1987; (15): 50–60.
8. According to Ogura (Reference 7), Hisayuki Shimazu (1695–1734) was the head of the Sashi Shimazu family, a branch family of the Shimazu feudal clan. Hisakiyo Shimazu (?–?) was the eldest son of Hisayuki Shimazu, but did not succeed his father because he had a cleft lip, which was repaired by Kore-eda and Nagai.
9. Ikeda S. Who Was the First to Administer General Anesthesia in Japan? *Bulletin of Anesthesia History* 2011; 29: 49–52.
10. Matsuki A. New Studies on the History of Anesthesiology (5) – A review of studies on the biography of Tokumei Takamine. *Masui* 2000; 49: 1169–73.
11. Matsuki A. New Studies on the History of Anesthesiology (6) – Re-evaluation of Basic Document Materials of Tokumei Takamine. *Masui* 2000; 49; 1285–9.

2   Hoyoku Takashi and Anesthesia−related Agents for Coaptation

Several anesthesia−related concoctions for coaptation are described in Hoyoku Takashi's (?–?) *Honetsugi Ryoji Chohoki* (Figure 2.2.1), which was published in 1746, approximately half a century before Hanaoka's first successful use of general anesthesia in 1804. The book is likely to be one of the first medical textbooks that discusses such agents written or edited by Japanese physicians and published in Japan. Thus, it is listed in the "Chronology of the History of Anesthesia in Japan."[1] Although Chinese medical books containing several formulae for anesthetic agents and their use had been imported to Japan before 1746, most practitioners could not apply them correctly because they were written in Chinese. Therefore, there was an urgent need, particularly among bonesetting practitioners, for a textbook on the subject written in Japanese. The foreword by the physician Takemasa Furubayashi (?–?) to the Takashi textbook gave an account of the challenging situation at that time. It reads as follows:

> Before long, Takashi is going to publish a textbook in Japanese, which reveals the art of coaptation. He ardently hopes to spread it among coaptation practitioners. The book would be benevolence to them.

Despite the importance of *Honetsugi Ryouji Chohoki*, there are few details on the life of Takashi. His given name was Shinkai; however, he had many

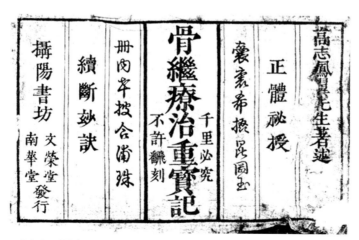

Figure 2.2.1   Title page of *Honetsugi Ryoji Chohoki*, published in 1746

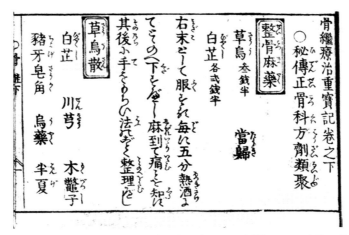

Figure 2.2.2 First page of the third volume of *Honetsugi Ryoji Chohoki*, describing "Seikotsu Mayaku" and "Sou san"

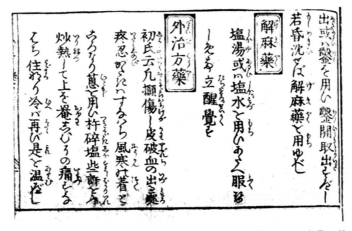

Figure 2.2.3 Third page of the third volume of *Honetsugi Ryoji Chohoki*, describing "Gemayaku"

pseudonyms, including Gento, Jikosai, and Hoyoku. It is known that at young age, Takashi studied Chinese under a Chinese Scholar, Ikan Hozumi (1693–1769) from Osaka. Hozumi attested that Takashi was a genius at Chinese. According to Shunseki Maeda (?–?), one of Takashi's protégés, Takashi was a man of versatility, an expert not only of Chinese but also of various specialties of medicine, including internal medicine, pediatrics,

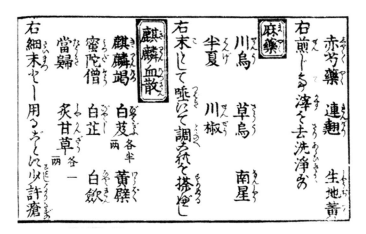

Figure 2.2.4   End of the third volume of *Honetsugi Ryoji Chohoki*, describing "Mayaku"

orthopedics, obstetrics, gynecology, ophthalmology, and acupuncture. Takashi was also said to be less than 30 years of age in 1746. It is known that Takashi wrote and edited more than 30 medical books, although except for *Honetsugi Ryoji Chohoki* and *Igaku Doshimon*, all of them remained unpublished.

For the three-volume *Honetsugi Ryoji Chohoki*, Takashi extracted accounts on orthopedic diseases and their treatments from various Chinese textbooks. The first volume contains Ikan Hozumi's foreword (1745); Takemasa Furubayashi's afterword (1745), Shunseki Maeda's afterword (1745), Shinkai Takashi's preface (1746), Contents of Volumes 1, 2, and 3, anatomy of the human body, basic principles of coaptation, and figures of the human body meridians. The second volume includes descriptions of orthopedic diseases from the head to the foot and their treatments, supplemented with numerous illustrations. It also provides oral directions for the drug use in bonesetting and 10 signs of incurable injuries. The appendix consists of the following: methods to remove metallic foreign bodies and the treatment of injuries from horse kicks, cow horning, and dog bites. The third volume is a collection of 103 formulae and directions for their use in the practice of coaptation. Again, most are likely derived from Chinese medical textbooks, with no original formulae developed by Takashi himself. Among them, four prescriptions are associated with anesthesia.

Three formulae out of four are mentioned in the first to third pages of the third volume (Figure 2.2.2–4). The first formula is called "Seikotsu Mayaku" (bonesetting anesthetic). The description reads as follows:

Seikotsu Mayaku
So–u (Caowu, *Aconitum carmichaeli Debx*), Toki (Dang–gui, *Angelica actiloba*), and Byakushi (Baizhi, *Angelica dahurica*)
    Grind them into powder and take with hot sake (wine) added one part of water. It produces numbness and patients feel no pain. Then, begin reduction manually as instructed in the book.
(Chinese name and botanical names in Latin in parenthesis. Unit abbreviated.)

    This anesthetic was to be orally administered when the reduction maneuver for a simple luxation or fracture was expected to be difficult because of pain. In cases of complicated injury or operative procedure, a more potent anesthetic called Sousan (Caowusan) was administered.
    The formula for Sousan (Caowusan) and directions for use are described in following section on "Seikotsu Mayaku."

Sousan (Caowusan)
Byakushi (Baizhi, *Angelica dahurica*), Senkyu (Chuan qiong, *Lingusticum chuanxiong*), Mokubetsushi (Mubiezi, *Momordica cohinchinensis*), Chogasokaku (Zhuya zaojiao, *Gleditsia sinensis*), Uyaku (Wuyao, *Lindela strychnifolia*), Hange (Ban xia, *Pinella ternata*), Shikimpi (Zijinpi, *Tripterygium hypoglaucum*), Totoki (Dudanggui, *Aralia cordata*), Sen–u (Chuanwu, *Aconitum carmichaeli*), Senjouikyo (Chuanshang huixiang, *Foeniculum vulgare*), Sou (Caowu, *Aconitum carmichaeli*), Mokko (Muxiang, *Saussurea lappa*)
    Grind them into powder. Administer it with sake (wine), and it causes numbness to feel no pain. In case of comminuted fractures, incise the wound with a knife and remove the bone fragments to reduce manually. Then apply a wood splint for fixing. The agent is also used to produce anesthesia when an arrowhead penetrating into the bone is difficult to extract. Remove it with iron forceps or excise the wound to extract it. When deep insensateness follows, give an antidote.
    (Chinese and botanical names in Latin in parenthesis. Unit abbreviated.)

    In this prescription, two types of aconitum ingredient are included: Sen–u (Chuanwu) and Sou (Caowu). By mixing the same types of ingredients from different districts, more potent effects were expected and with fewer side effects. Most ingredients were also included in the prescriptions of Hanai and Onishi,[2] and Hanaoka is said to have modified their prescriptions to develop his own "Mafutsusan."

The third formula is an antidote called "Gemayaku" consisting of salt water, sometimes hot. When the patient was still comatose after surgery because of a general anesthetic, salt water was given.

The fourth prescription is found on page 96 of the third volume and is called "Mayaku," meaning anesthetics or analgesics. It reads as follows:

Mayaku
Sen-u (Chuanwu, *Aconitum carmichaeli Debx.*), Sou (Caowu, *Aconitum carmichaeli Debx.*), Nansei (Nanxing, *Arisaema consanguneum*), Hange (Banxia, *Pinella ternata*), Sensho (Chuanjiao, *Zanthoxylum*)
Grind them into powder. Knead with saliva and apply it to the incision.
(Chinese name and botanical names in Latin in parenthesis. Unit abbreviated.)

It is apparent that "Mayaku" is a topical anesthetic since the phrase "Knead with saliva" is included in the account. Among the five ingredients included, Sen-u and Sou have potent topical analgesic properties because both contain aconitum.

These four formulae are likely to have been reproduced from the Chinese medical textbook *Yangke Zhengchi Zhuosheng* written by Wang Ken-tang (1549–1613) and published in 1608, as there are no significant differences in ingredients, formulae, or accounts (except for language). Among the four formulae, Caowusan dates back to *Shiyi Dexiao Fang*, published in 1345; however, it should be noted that Caowusan in *Shiyi Dexiao Fang* includes a component of datura as an extra ingredient, which was also the main ingredient of Hanaoka's "Mafutsusan."

According to "*Mayaku Ko*" written by Shutei Nakagawa (1773–1850), a close junior colleague of Hanaoka, he observed Hanaoka's successful experiments with general anesthetics in more than 10 human volunteers before 1796, which strongly suggests that Nakagawa would have shared information on general anesthetics with Hanaoka.[3,4] Nakagawa's manuscript contains 16 concoctions of general anesthetics, 3 topical analgesics, and an antidote. Among them, are Caowusan, Hanai's formula, and Onishi's formula.[2] Caowusan is the original formula of Hanai and Onishi. The manuscript also refers to Hanaoka's general anesthetic, which is modified from Hanai's or Onishi's prescriptions.

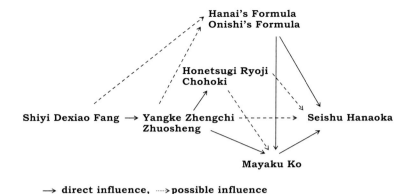

Figure 2.2.5　Factors (books and formulae) influencing Hanaoka's development of general anesthetic

The four formulae appearing in Takashi's book are also found in "*Mayaku Ko*." However, Nakagawa likely referred to *Yangke Zhengchi Zhuosheng* through Takashi's book and extracted them directly because all are in Chinese. As mentioned, it is reasonable to speculate that Nakagawa would have shared his knowledge of general anesthetics with Hanaoka because the latter had devoted himself to developing an effective general anesthetic. Although there is no direct proof that Hanaoka read "*Mayaku Ko*," *Honetsugi Ryoji Chohoki*, or *Yangke Zhengchi Zhuosheng*, it is likely that he was influenced by these books and modified the formulae of Hanai and Onishi to develope his own anesthetic "Mafutsusan." Several factors influencing Hanaoka are illustrated in Figure 2.2.5.

References and Remarks

1. Matsuki A. *A Short History of Anesthesia in Japan*. Hirosaki, Hirosaki University Press, 2013. p.211.
2. Matsuki A. *Seishu Hanaoka and His Medicine – A Japanese Pioneer of Anesthesia and Surgery –*. (2nd ed.) Hirosaki, Hirosaki University Press, 2011. p.55–6.
3. Reference 2. p.53–5.
4. Reference 1. p.22–6.

3 Sadakichi Iwanaga from Kyoto–Another of Hanaoka's Preceptors of Surgery

It is important when considering the history of anesthesia in Japan to appreciate the academic genealogy of Naomichi Hanaoka (thereafter referred to as Naomichi to avoid misunderstanding, 1722–1785) and Seishu Hanaoka (referred as Seishu, 1760–1835), the eldest son of Naomichi. According to Kure,[1] two physicians were Seishu's preceptors of surgery. One is his father Naomichi and the other is Kenryu Yamato (1750–1827). Naomichi had studied Dutch-style surgery under Bangen Iwanaga (referred to as Bangen, 1673–1729) in Osaka; though when and for how long Naomichi apprenticed with Bangen remain unclear. Seishu learned the practice of medicine from Naomichi, who was his only teacher until he traveled to Kyoto as there was no other preceptor near to his native village.

In 1782, at the age of 22, Seishu visited Kyoto to further study medicine. It was the first long distance trip he took. In Kyoto, Seishu initially learned liberal arts for approximately one and a half years and then learned internal medicine and surgery under various teachers for the remaining one and a half years. One of his teachers was Kenryu Yamato, who practiced Dutch-style surgery.[2] Unfortunately, Yamato's detailed career and academic pedigree remain unclear. In 1966, Otsuka[3] examined a manuscript titled "*Joka Sentei*" by Shutei Nakagawa and reported that a surgeon named Iwanaga of Kyoto was one of the preceptors of Seishu. In response to Otsuka's article, Nakano[4] described a commentary following Otsuka's paper that there were two branches of the Iwanaga family from Osaka, one was the Bangen family and the other was the Gensho (younger brother of Bangen) family. Nakano uncovered the names and death dates of four consecutive generations of the Gensho family but did not provide any information on the Bangen family.

Naomichi's preceptor is unlikely to have been Bangen because Naomichi was born in 1722, and according to the temple record (below) Bangen died in 1729. This strongly suggests that Naomichi studied surgery from "Bangen, Jr." because it was common at that time in Japan that for a son to succeed his father's name in a physician's family. I examined the burial records of Jokoji Temple,[5] the Bangen family's temple, and found a total of five posthumous names of the family members, including that of Bangen, and produced a pedigree of the Bangen Iwanaga family to identify the preceptor of Naomichi, as shown in Figure 2.3.1.[6] Given names are in parentheses. A solid line indicates the identified relationship, and a dotted line indicates a possible

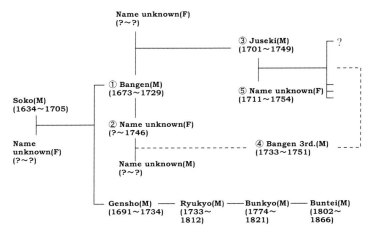

Figure 2.3.1 Pedigree of the Iwanaga family from Osaka. The pedigree of the Gensho family according to Nakano's paper.

relationship.

The five members of the Bangen family read as follows: (Death date; Posthumous name; Name, including childhood name; and Age in years according to the Japanese system.)

① July 21, 14th Year of Kyoho (1729) Shuzen Bangen Iwanaga 57 years old

② November 7, 3rd Year of Enkyo (1746) Myozen Mother-in-law of Juseki, Wife of Bangen

③ April 18, 2nd Year of Kan-en (1749) Soju Juseki Iwanaga 49 years old

④ December 27, 1st Year of Horeki (1751) Sogen A young brother of Iwanaga, Bangen 3rd, Childhood name Itsuro

⑤ July 24, 4th Year of Horeki (1754) Myoju Wife of Juseki Iwanaga 44 years old

According to this pedigree, Bangen (①, the elder) died in 1729 and therefore could not have been the preceptor of Naomichi. Juseki ③ was a son of Bangen and his ex-wife because ② (Name unknown) was the mother–in–law of Juseki. Although Juseki is not described as "Bangen Jr.," it is most likely that Juseki succeeded Bangen ① and declared himself Bangen Jr. Bangen 3rd. ④ was not a son of Bangen ①; he was born 4 years after Bangen's death. Considering the burial record description of "A young brother of Iwanaga," he is likely to be Bangen's second wife's ② son by a previous marriage. There is another possibility that Bangen 3rd. ④ could be the second son of Juseki ③ because Bangen 3rd. was also described as "Bangen 3rd. and a younger brother of Bangen" in the burial records. Based on this description, he would have succeeded Juseki or "Bangen Jr." since his elder brother or the eldest son of Bangen had died earlier. However, this is less likely because the posthumous name of Bangen's eldest son is not detected in the burial records.

If Naomichi had visited Osaka at the age of 20–25 years, it would have been in a period between1745–1749, when Juseki ③ was alive. Thus, Juseki was most likely the mentor of Naomichi. There are no names of the Gensho family in the burial records of the Jokoji Temple because their family temples were different.

According to a manuscript titled "*Nihon Ifu*"[7] by Kondai Utsuki (1779–1848), a family called "Iwanaga" lived in Kyoto. They were relatives of Bangen from Osaka. The description reads as follows:

> Samon Iwanaga. Another surname is Sugawara. Specialized in surgery and renowned at that times in Kyoto. His son was Sadakichi, another name is Ryotoku, his alias is Kodo, and the pseudonym is Bokusai. He succeeded his father and specialized in surgery. No children as successors.

Although the exact years of birth and death of Samon remain unknown, he is said to have been active in the year of Kyoho or a period between 1716–1735, half a century before Seishu visited Kyoto to study medicine in the 1780s. Thus, Samon was unlikely to be Seishu's preceptor. Sadakichi, the second–generation member, is identified as Seishu's teacher because there was no other Iwanaga family in Kyoto. Sadakichi's possible active period covers the 3 years between 1782–1785 when Seishu stayed in Kyoto.

According to Kure[1] and Nakano[8], Bangen moved to Osaka from Nagasaki in the year of Shotoku or between 1711–1715. Soko Iwanaga (1634–1705) was likely Bangen's father. He was a physician from Nagasaki and a disciple of Gensho Mukai (1609–1659).[9–11] Mukai was a Western–style physician as well as a Confucian physician. In the 1650s he learned "red–head–style" (Western) external medicine from several physicians and surgeons who

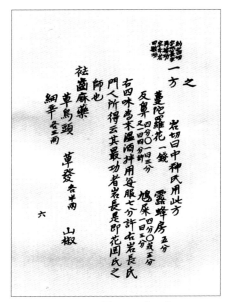
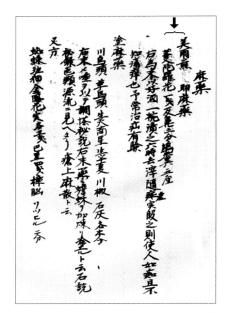

Figure 2.3.2 Formula that a disciple of Iwanaga unfolded (Taken from "*Mayaku Ko*")

Figure 2.3.3 Formula of "Bilzenkruid" (Taken from "*Zoku Kimpo Roku*) With kind permission from the Kyo-u Library.

belonged to the Dutch factory in Dejima, one of them was Hans Jurian Hancke (?–?).[12]

According to Shutei Nakagawa's "*Mayaku Ko*," Iwanaga from Kyoto did not disclose the general anesthetic that he used in surgery.[13] This Iwanaga is likely to have been Seishu's preceptor Sadakichi considering the context of the manuscript. "*Mayaku Ko*" also describes a formula for a general anesthetic containing four ingredients, that one of Iwanaga's disciples divulged. It reads as follows:

> Mandarage (datura), Rohobo (beehive), Hambi (pit viper, *Agkistrodon blomhoffi*), and Kyushi (pigeon's excrements)
> (unit abbreviated) (Figure 2.3.2)

A similar formula is found in the first part of "Mayaku (Anesthetics)" in the manuscript "*Zoku Kimpo Roku*" edited by Seishu,[14] and the formula is titled "Birusen" or "Anesthetic" as shown in Figure 2.3.3.

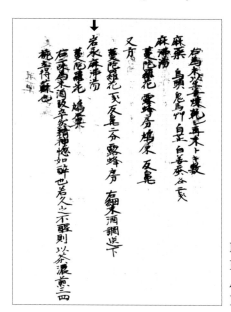

Figure 2.3.4 Formula of "Iwanaga Mafutsu To" (Taken from "*Zoku Kimpo Roku*) With kind permission from the Kyo–u Library.

"Birusen" or "Anesthetic"
Mandarage (datura), Hambi (pit viper, *Agkistrodon blomhoffi*), and Kyushi (pigeon's excrements)   (unit abbreviated)

"Birusen" is a Chinese transcription of "bilzen," an abbreviation of the Dutch word "bilzenkruid," suggesting that the formula originated from Dutch style medicine and not from traditional Chinese medicine. "*Zoku Kimpo Roku*" also mentions a prescription called "Iwanaga's Mafutsuto" consisting of only two ingredients, Mandarage (datura) and Kyushi (pigeon's excrements), as illustrated in Figure 2.3.4. Among these three prescriptions, the last formula is the simplest and is likely based on an original concoction handed down from Dutch physicians at Dejima because formulae generally become more complex with time. In addition, "Hambi," an ingredient indigenous to Japan, was likely added later. In any case, it is likely that Hanaoka had learned from Sadakichi Iwanaga something about the surgical treatment of breast cancer and the general anesthetic vital for achieving Hanaoka's goal.

References and Remarks

1. Kure S. *Seishu Hanaoka and His Surgery.* Tokyo, Tohodo, 1923. p.5–6, 13–5.
2. Matsuki A. *Seishu Hanaoka and His Medicine – A Japanese Pioner of Anesthesia and Surgery – .* (2nd ed.) Hirosaki, Hirosaki University Press, 2011. p.23–7.
3. Otsuka K. A View that Shutei Nakagawa is a disciple of Seishu Hanaoka is not correct. *Itan* (reissue series) 1966; (33): 17–21.
4. Nakano M. On the Iwanaga Family. *Itan* (reissue series) 1966; (33): 21.
5. The temple was located in Saito–cho, Osaka City, but moved to Kotobukicho, Suita City about 50 years ago.
6. Matsuki A. *New Development in the Study of Seishu Hanaoka.* Tokyo, Shinkokoeki Ishoshuppanbu, 2013. p.102.
7. The manuscript is in the possession of The University of Tokyo Library. Gakken Collection (V10: 336)
8. Nakano M. Bangen Iwanaga. In: The Japan–Netherlands Institute. ed. *Dictionary of the History of Western Studies.* Tokyo, Yushodo, 1984. p.70–1.
9. Michel W. On the Medical Staff of the Dutch Factories in Hirado and Nagasaki during the 17th Century. *J. Japan Society Medical History* 1995; 41: 403–20.
10. Michel W. On the Manuscript "Recipes of Dutch Surgery" (Oranda geka seiden) and the Cofusian Scholar Mukai Genshō. *Hikaku shakai bunka* 1996; (2): 75–9.
11. Michel W. On Early Red–head–style External Medicine and the Confucian Physician Mukai Genshō. *J. Japan Society Medical History* 2010; 56: 367–85.
12. Michel W. On the Dejima factory surgeon Hans Jurian Hancko. *Gengo bunka ronkyu* (*Kyushu University*) 1996; (7): 83–96.
13. Matsuki A. *A Short History of Anesthesia in Japan.* p.24–5.
14. "*Zoku Kimpo Roku*" is in the possession of Kyo–u Library of Takeda Science Foundation. (2 Vols., Kyo. 5741)

4   Seishu Hanaoka's Philosophy of "Safety and Challenge"

This section is mainly based on a keynote lecture delivered at the opening ceremony of the 13th Asian and Australasian Congress of Anaesthesiologists held in Fukuoka, Japan, in 2010. Because several new facts pertaining to Seishu Hanaoka have emerged in the last 6 years, necessary revisions have been made.

Figure 2.4.1 is a portrait of Hanaoka in formal attire as a feudal physician of the Kishu Domain (presently Wakayama Prefecture). Red crests, suggesting a surgeon's knot, are observed on his half–coat. In 1804, Hanaoka gave general anesthesia to a woman named Kan Aiya for the extirpation of breast cancer. This is considered the first use of general anesthesia in the world. To be identified as "the first in the world," six criteria must be satisfied: the name of the patient, the name of the surgeon, the sort of surgery, the date

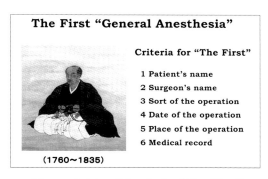

Figure 2.4.1   Criteria for "The First"

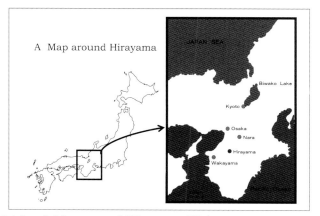

Figure 2.4.2   A Map around Hirayama, Wakayama Prefecture

"Miscellaneous Travel Notes" (1764)

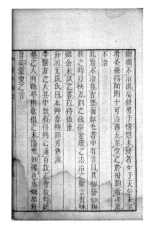 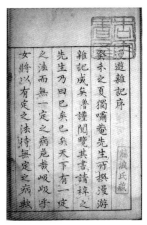

Figure 2.4.3   "Man-yu zakki"

"Breast cancer is incurable since early times. In a western medical textbook, they state the breast cancer can be excised surgically when the tumor is like an apricot seed in the initial stage. As I have not tried the excision yet, I mention this here, expecting future trial by young physicians."

Figure 2.4.4   Nagatomi's Description of Breast Cancer

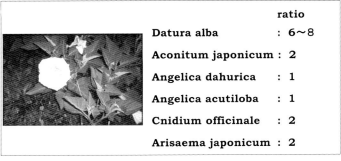

	ratio
Datura alba	: 6〜8
Aconitum japonicum	: 2
Angelica dahurica	: 1
Angelica acutiloba	: 1
Cnidium officinale	: 2
Arisaema japonicum	: 2

Figure 2.4.5   Herbal Mixture of "Mafutsusan"

of the surgery, and the place where the surgery was performed must be known. In addition, a reliable medical record must exist. This case meets all six of these conditions.[1]

A simple map of the region around the village of Hirayama, Hanaoka's birthplace, is shown in Figure 2.4.2. The village is 20 km northeast of Wakayama City and approximately 100 km from Kyoto in a straight line. Hanaoka was the eldest son of the village doctor. He grew up in the village and learned medicine privately from his father. In 1782, at the age of 22 years, he went to Kyoto to study medicine because Kyoto was then a major center for medical studies. Because his family was not rich, he was unable to afford a trip to Nagasaki or Edo (presently Tokyo), other centers of medical study in Japan at that time. He stayed in Kyoto for 3 years, during which he arduously studied liberal arts and Western style surgery as well as traditional Chinese medicine under various masters.[2]

During his stay in Kyoto, Hanaoka read "*Man–yu zakki*" (Figure 2.4.3) or "Miscellaneous Travel Notes" by Dokushoan Nagatomi (1732–1766), a famous physician from the Choshu Domain (presently Yamaguchi Prefecture), and was deeply impressed by a paragraph in the book.[3] The preface of the book is shown on the right side of Figure 2.4.3, and the paragraph that particularly impressed Hanaoka is shown on the left (the 4th to 6th lines from right). An English translation is shown in Figure 2.4.4.

Hanaoka eventually developed the oral general anesthetic "Mafutsusan." The left side of Figure 2.4.5 depicts Datura alba, referred to as "Korean morning glory" in Japan, which resembles (but not the same as) the species Datura alba Nees that Hanaoka used. The word "Korean" in this context means "exotic." The herbal mixture "Mafutsusan" is on the right of this figure. Datura is the main ingredient.

After approximately 20 years of experimentation, Hanaoka came to the conclusion that a combination of datura and aconite is the best combination for producing surgical anesthesia. It is said that his mother Otsugi and his wife Ka–e participated in the experiments; however, no substantial proof is extant and the details of their contributions remain unknown.[3]

Figure 2.4.6 illustrates the first part of the list of breast cancer patients treated, revealing that Hanaoka began treating breast cancer in January 1804. The first three patients refused surgery because they had never heard of a surgical excision under general anesthesia, which they feared. However, the fourth patient Kan Aiya strongly requested that Hanaoka perform surgery on her, making her the first person to be operated on under general anesthesia. According to the list, the date was October 16; however, her surgery was

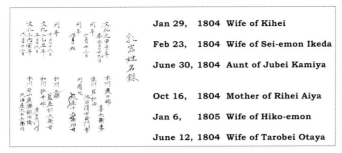

Jan 29, 1804	Wife of Kihei
Feb 23, 1804	Wife of Sei-emon Ikeda
June 30, 1804	Aunt of Jubei Kamiya
Oct 16, 1804	Mother of Rihei Aiya
Jan 6, 1805	Wife of Hiko-emon
June 12, 1804	Wife of Tarobei Otaya

Figure 2.4.6 The List of Breast Cancer Patients

The Manuscript of The First Case

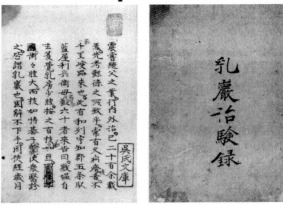

Figure 2.4.7 The Manuscript titled "*Nyugan Chiken Roku*"

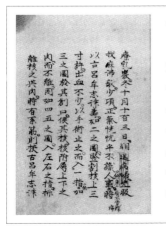

"On the morning of Oct 13th, I gave her my Mahutsu-san. After a while, she became drowsy, then lost consciousness. I made an incision above the tumor like Fig 2. She bled a lot. "

Figure 2.4.8 Description of Kan's Operation in "*Nyugan Chiken Roku*"

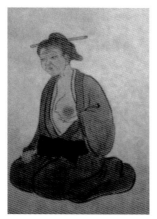 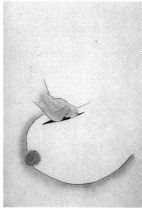

Figure 2.4.9   Illustrations of Kan Aiya and An Incision of the Left Breast

performed on October 13, 1804 (October 16 was the day she was registered in the list). It took 40 days to improve her preoperative condition because she had suffered from beriberi and asthma.[4,5]

Figure 2.4.7 depicts the title page (right side of the figure) and the first page (the left side) of the medical record or manuscript titled "*Nyugan Chiken Roku*" describing this first surgical case. It was written by one of Hanaoka's disciples, who appeared to have been his (as yet unidentified) assistant.[6] It is thought that Hanaoka asked him to transcribe this record from dictation.

The left side of Figure 2.4.8 illustrates the fifth leaf (11th page) of the manuscript, where there is a description (the first to third lines) of the patient Kan given general anesthesia. The English translation would be as follows: "On the morning of October 13, I gave her my Mafutsusan. After a while, she became drowsy and then lost consciousness. I made an incision above the tumor like Figure 2. She bled a lot."

Figure 2.4.9 depicts reproductions of the original Figures 1 and 2. The original Figure 1 is a picture of the patient Kan, and the original Figure 2 shows that Hanaoka was performing a tumor excision but not a mastectomy.

Kan's burial record at Komodoji Temple in Gojo City, Nara Prefecture, shown on the left side of Figure 2.4.10 indicates that she died on February 26, 1805, four and half a months after the surgery. "Shungetsu Chiryo Shinjo" is her posthumous name, and "Kitano-machi" is her dwelling place. Her death was probably not expected by Hanaoka and must have had a grave impact on him.

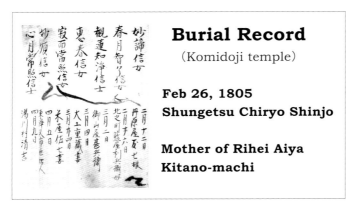

Burial Record
(Komidoji temple)

Feb 26, 1805
Shungetsu Chiryo Shinjo

Mother of Rihei Aiya
Kitano-machi

Figure 2.4.10 Burial Record of Kan Aiya

Case No	Date of Surgery	Interval
1	Oct 13, 1804	2.5 months
2	Jan 6, 1805	
	Feb 26 Kan died	16 months
3	Apr 8, 1806	2 months
4	Jun 12, 1806	

Figure 2.4.11 Interval between The First Four Surgical Cases
(Intercalary month of August is in 1805.)

Year	No of Disciples
1804	10
Oct 13 Kan's operation	
1805	0
Feb 26 Kan died	
1806	14
1807	4

Figure 2.4.12 Numbers of Disciples Entered Hanaoka's School between 1804 and 1807

Figure 2.4.11 shows the intervals between the first four breast cancer surgeries. There was a long interval of 16 months between the second and third cases, the period during which Kan died. Such a long interval is not observed thereafter, which suggests that Hanaoka was distressed by Kan's early and unexpected death and suspected that it had been caused by his method of surgery. Consequently, he may have decided to not perform subsequent breast cancer surgeries until he re-examined his procedures.

Hanaoka's cautiousness can be verified by the number of the disciples accepted in his school "Shunrinken" (Figure 2.4.12). No one was admitted in 1805, the year Kan died, while every other year Hanaoka accepted four to ten students. The year 1805 was the only year since 1801 when no one was admitted, which suggests that Hanaoka refused to accept students in that year to devote his time to reassessing his surgical procedure.[7] However, he was unable to find deficiencies in the procedure and resumed his surgical treatments in April 1806. He also began enrolling new students sometime in 1806.

Hanaoka performed breast cancer surgery on more than 140 patients.[8] Figure 2.4.13 shows one of the scrolls illustrating various rare diseases also treated by Hanaoka. The names and addresses of the patients were written but they are too small to be seen. Patients with various diseases came to him, mostly from southwestern Japan because no other surgeon could cure them at the time.[9]

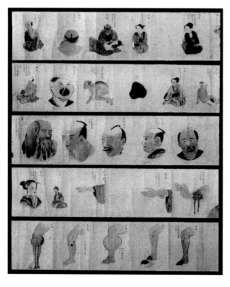

Figure 2.4.13 Illustrations of Rare Diseases Treated by Hanaoka (1838)

> **Hanaoka's Philosophy of "Safety and Challenge"**
>
> **Safety**
>
> : Waited 40 days to improve Kan's physical condition
>
> : Postponed for 15 months to resume the ensuing breast cancer operations
>
> **Challenge**
>
> : Gave " the first " clinical anesthetic
>
> : Performed various surgical operations

Figure 2.4.14 Hanaoka's Philosophy

Hanaoka was very concerned for the safety of his patients, and was in no hurry to perform the first breast cancer surgery. Indeed, he tended to Kan for 40 days prior to the operation. He postponed any further breast cancer surgeries for 15 months after her death. These actions clearly demonstrate Hanaoka's philosophy of "Safety" in care of a patient. He succeeded in developing the general anesthetic "Mafutsusan" after 20 years of experimentation. He also treated various diseases that other surgeons could not, which exemplifies his philosophy of "Challenge." These actions demonstrate his dual philosophy of "Safety and Challenge" (Figure 2.4.14).[10]

In Hanaoka's era, Japan subscribed to a policy of national isolation, and Japanese medical information was disseminated to foreign countries only rarely through Nagasaki, the single open door to Western countries. Therefore, Hanaoka's method had little chance of influencing Western medicine in the short term. Regardless, Hanaoka's medical and surgical treatments spread widely throughout Japan and greatly contributed to the rapid acceptance of modern Western surgery in the ensuing period.

References and Remarks

1. Matsuki A. *Seishu Hanaoka and His Medicine – A Japanese Pioneer of Anesthesia and Surgery –*. (2nd ed.) p.73–4.
   In this section, the sixth condition "the place where the surgery was performed" was newly added.
2. Reference 1. p.13–5.

3. Reference 1. p.52–3.
4. Reference 1. p.73–4.
5. Matsuki A. *A Short History of Anesthesia in Japan.* p.35–40.
6. Reference 1. p.83–91.
7. Reference 1. p.156.
8. Reference 1. p.101–8.
9. There are many manuscripts that illustrate rare diseases for which Hanaoka and his disciples performed operations. For details, see the following reference.
   Matsuki A. *New Development in the Study of Seishu Hanaoka.* p.171–249.
10. For another aspect of Hanaoka's philosophy, see Reference1. p.172–6.

5   Introduction of Inhaled Anesthesia to Batavia and Japan

The circumstances through which chloroform and ether were introduced to Batavia (presently Jakarta) and then to Japan are briefly mentioned in the explanations for Slide 13 and 14 in Chapter 1 of this book. A more detailed discussion is provided in this section.

The anesthetic properties of chloroform were discovered in November 4, 1847 by James Young Simpson (1811–1870)[1-3] of Edinburgh, Scotland, who was quick to apply it in clinical practice. Only 6 days later, on November 10, he read the first report on its clinical use to the Edinburgh Medical and Chirurgical Society. These events occurred within 13 months after the public demonstration of ether anesthesia in 1846 by William T. G. Morton (1819–1868) in Boston. Consequently, information on the use of chloroform anesthesia spread around the world approximately a year later than that of ether anesthesia, with the exception of Japan.[4]

At that time, Japan still subscribed to a national isolation policy, and Nagasaki was the only place where trade took place with foreign countries. The Netherlands was the only western country allowed to trade with Japan through the Dutch East India Factory located at Dejima, Nagasaki. Consequently, information about Western civilization, including the medical sciences, was brought to Japan from the Netherlands through the Dutch East India government in Batavia and then to Japan through the factory, which was an agency of the government in Japan. Thus, information on ether and chloroform anesthesia was conveyed from the Netherlands to Nagasaki via the government in Batavia. Therefore, to understand the introduction of these agents in Japan, it is necessary to know the circumstances under which both drugs were first brought to Batavia.

According to previous investigations,[5,6] Otto G. J. Mohnike, a German physician and medical attaché to the factory at Dejima, was the first to convey information on inhaled anesthesia to Japan when he described the new technique to Soken Narabayashi, a physician from the Saga Domain (Saga Prefecture) in August 1848. The inhaled anesthetic that Mohnike described was not ether but chloroform, although information on ether anesthesia was brought to Japan a year later in June 1849 when a copy of the Dutch edition of J. Schlesinger's book on ether anesthesia was imported. Seikei Sugita published a Japanese translation in March 1850.[7] Therefore, the introduction of the concept of inhaled anesthetics to Japan is likely to be the only exceptional case in the world in which information on chloroform anesthesia preceded that on ether anesthesia.

The reason for this exception can be explained as follows: In 1847, ether anesthesia was introduced to Batavia, the capital of Dutch East India. Physicians of the Batavia Hospital first conducted experiments with ether in frogs, fish, sparrows, rabbits, and dogs. After this series of animal experiments, a physician named Schreuder unsuccessfully tried to produce clinical anesthesia in several surgical patients. In addition, he tested ether on himself twice but found it to cause headache and dizziness without sedative effects. In 1848, Dr. Wassink at the Simpang Hospital, Surabaya, Dutch East India, attempted to administer ether to seven surgical patients; however, he too failed to provide satisfactory anesthesia. In the early months of 1848, chloroform was also introduced to them. Dr. Bleeker of the Batavia Hospital administered chloroform to a patient for amputation of the lower leg, and the accompanying pain was much alleviated. Dr. Wassink also administered chloroform during leg amputation to three patients, and the effects of the agent were almost satisfactory. Although "excitements" were observed during anesthesia, they were "nothing compared with those experienced formerly in similar cases."[8,9] It is likely that physicians of Dutch East India judged chloroform as a useful anesthetic but ether as ineffective as evidenced by the fact that Schreuder reported his experiences with chloroform anesthesia, but not ether anesthesia.[10]

Dr. Mohnike, another physician at the Batavia Hospital, learned of these anesthetic cases and the greater efficacy of chloroform in the clinical setting. With this in mind, he visited Japan in June 1848. Two months later, in August 1848, Mohnike informed Soken Narabayashi of "chloroform analgesia," but not of "chloroform anesthesia." This implies that at Batavia, Mohnike would have learned of chloroform inhalation, which did not cause complete loss of consciousness.

In 1851, Shinsuke Maeda (1821–1918), a feudal physician from the Kagoshima Domain (Kagoshima Prefecture), wrote a manuscript titled "*A Dialogue with Mohnike*" (tentative title) in which Mohnike's brief comments on stethoscope, ether anesthesia, anal prolapse, leprosy, epilepsy, and nocturnal enuresis were transcribed. An account titled "ether inhalation" reads as follows:

> In some patients, inhalation of ether not only produces no insensateness but also causes a retardation of incisional wound healing, leading to a serious postoperative result. Because of these reasons, physicians never use the agent in Western countries. In surgical operations, it is strongly

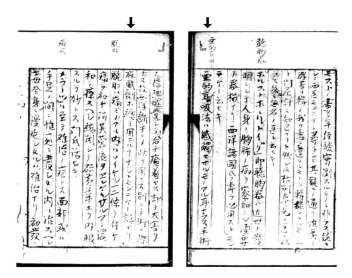

Figure 2.5.1 An account of ether anesthesia recorded on August 21, 1851. Right side is page 1 and the left side page 2. With kind permission from the University of Tokyo Library.

recommended to use no anesthetics and hypnotics. (Figure 2.5.1)

This description suggests that Mohnike considered the use of ether anesthesia useless and even contraindicated in surgeries. Although he introduced the concept of chloroform analgesia to Japan, he brought neither chloroform nor ether with him. Thus, there is no substantial proof that he performed surgery using general anesthesia. The medical attachés of the factory who succeeded him were unlikely to have a strong interest in general anesthesia, and none produced relevant documents on the subject until Pompe van Meerdervoort (1829–1908, referred to as Pompe).

Pompe[11] visited Japan as a member of the second mission to the Naval Training Center in Nagasaki and stayed there from August 1857 to November 1862, where he taught Japanese medical students. It is apparent that he brought chloroform to Japan, but exactly when remains unknown. However, he was not contemplating its use for surgical anesthesia in a clinical setting. It was in Edo (Tokyo) in June 1861 where Gemboku Ito (1800–1871), one of Pompe's disciples, administered chloroform anesthesia to a male patient named Yoshijiro Sakuragawa (?–?) to amputate Sakuragawa's gangrenous right foot. Ito used the agent that Pompe had brought or imported. This is

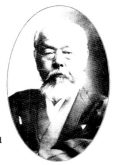

Figure 2.5.2 Kenzo Yoshida (1848 - 1918). Taken from *Temboku Essays* published in 1924.

the first documented case of chloroform anesthesia in Japan,[12] 13 years after information of the anesthetic properties of chloroform had been reached Japan by Mohnike.

It was William Willis (1837–1894), an English physician to the British consulate to Japan at Yokohama, who had the greatest impact on Japanese surgeons by practicing chloroform anesthesia. He treated soldiers from the Satsuma Domain injured at the battles of Toba and Fushimi in Kyoto and other battles of the Boshin War (1868–1869).[13] The British consulate supported the Satsuma and Tosa (presently Kochi Prefecture) Domains, two of the allied forces against the Tokugawa shogunate; therefore, Willis took care of the wounded of these domains. His practice of chloroform anesthesia impressed Japanese surgeons, particularly because of its prompt onset.

Kenzo Yoshida (1848–1918) (Figure 2.5.2)[14] was a Japanese surgeon from the Geishu Domain (presently Hiroshima Prefecture) who observed chloroform anesthesia during Willis' surgeries at the Shokokuji Temple, Kyoto, where a field hospital of the Satsuma Domain was located. Yoshida had learned Dutch style medicine from Yusei Kodama (?–1897), a physician of Arida Village near Yoshida's home village in the Geishu Domain. Observing Willis' practice of chloroform anesthesia, Yoshida was impressed by its rapid effects and soon successfully administered chloroform anesthesia to a male patient named Nakamura, who had attempted "hara-kiri," to squeeze the protruded intestines back into the abdominal cavity and suture the abdominal wall. The patient completely recovered from the surgery within a month but was later executed as a criminal. Later, Yoshida joined the Department of the Navy as a surgeon and visited London in 1872 to study medicine at University College, London, for 6 years.

Gen-yu Hirota (1831–1895) (Figure 2.5.3)[15,16] was another Japanese surgeon who observed Willis' practice of chloroform anesthesia. He was a

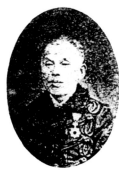

Figure 2.5.3 Gen-yu Hirota (1831 - 1895). Taken from Shiba's paper (Reference 15)

feudal physician from the Tosa Domain and learned Dutch style medicine in 1850 under Koan Ogata (1810–1863) in Osaka. The following year, he entered Gassuido School in Osaka, the branch of Hanaoka's Shunrinken school at Hirayama in the Kishu Domain. How long he studied at Gassuido remains unknown. He joined the Boshin War as a military surgeon of the Tosa Domain and was active in treating casualties. On the intercalary month April 10, 1868, at the battle of Mibu (Tochigi Prefecture), he administered chloroform anesthesia to a soldier named Taisuke Yoshikawa for amputation of his upper arm, although from whom he learned and how to administer the drug remain unknown. He also used the agent on May 3 in Edo for index finger amputation of a soldier named Chozaburo Oda. Although documented cases of chloroform anesthesia are few, these cases suggest that its use began to spread among Japanese surgeons during the Boshin War, primarily because of its easy administration and rapid onset. Hirota would be the third Japanese surgeon to practice the use of chloroform anesthesia.

A copy of the Dutch edition of J. Schlesinger's book on ether anesthesia was imported in 1849 and translated into Japanese and published by Seikei Sugita in March 1850, thus information on inhaled anesthesia with ether was transmitted to Japan by March 1850. Nevertheless, there is no proof that either Mohnike or Pompe brought the agent with them. In fact, based on experiences in Dutch East India, it is possible that they thought anesthetic ether to be ineffective for clinical anesthesia. In addition, there is no documented evidence of a Japanese physician requesting ether from the Dutch factory.

Soda[17] reported that Seikei Sugita had used ether anesthesia in two cases in 1855 but did not indicate the source document. Accordingly, I wrote in a previous book: "Thus, Sugita's administration of ether anesthesia in 1855 is not substantiated by any reliable document and remains hearsay."[18]

Thereafter, I carefully examined possible documents relating to this issue and finally found an article by Susumu Sato (1845–1921)[19] of the Juntendo Hospital in which Sugita's use of ether anesthesia is described.

According to the article, Sugita attempted, in either the 2nd or 3rd year of Ansei (1855 or 1856), to perform a surgery for repair of a burn scar on the hand of one of his disciples. Sugita used ether prepared in Edo by the chemist Ryuho Shima (1807–1873). After inhaling the agent from a bottle, the patient fell into a transient stupor but soon regained consciousness before the surgery. The patient again breathed the agent; however, no expected effects were obtained. Thus, the procedure is considered to have been conducted without effective anesthesia. The impurity of the ether synthesized by Shina is one possible reason for this. Sugita also tried to conduct a breast tumor excision using ether anesthesia; a number of physicians came to observe the surgery. Although the woman inhaled ether vapor, she did not lose consciousness because she was nervous and became excited to see many onlookers, and the surgery appears to have been canceled. Therefore, there is no documented case of successful ether anesthesia in the Edo era between the publication of Sugita's translation in 1850 and the last year of the Edo era in 1868.

References and Remarks

1. Keys TE. *The History of Surgical Anesthesia*. New York, Schuman's, 1945. p.33–5.
2. Duncum BM. *The Development of Inhalation Anaesthesia*. London, Oxford University Press,1947. p.167–81.
3. Rushman GB, Davies NJH, and Atkinson RS. *A Short History of Anaesthesia. The First 150 Years*. Oxford, Butterworth–Heinemann, 1996. p.24–6.
4. Reference 3. p.16–8.
5. Matsuki A. *A New Study on the History of Anesthesiology in Japan*. Tokyo, Kokuseido Shuppan, 2010. p.90–3.
6. Matsuki A. *A Short History of Anesthesia in Japan*. p.81–4.
7. Reference 6. p.73–81.
8. Schoute D. *De Geneeskunde in Nederlandisch– Indie gedurende de negentiende eeuw*. Batavia, G.Kolff, 1936. p.257.
9. Schoute D. *Occidental therapeutics in the Netherlands East Indies during three Centuries of Netherlands Settlement* (*1600–1900*). Batavia, G.Kolff, 1937. p.147.
10. Schroeuder HA. Anesthesie door chloroform–inademing. Tijdschr. Veren. T. Bevord. D. *Geneesk. Wetensche. Nederl. Indie, Batav.* 1852; i: 499–517.
11. Aikawa T. *Medicine at Dejima*. Nagasaki, Nagasaki Bunkensha, 2012. p.112–

26.
12. Matsuki A. *A Short History of Anesthesia in Japan*. p.84–5.
13. ibid. p.90–4.
14. Yoshida K. *Reminiscences, Temboku Essays*. Osaka, Yoshida K., 1924. p.17–8.
15. Shiba T. Reports on Disciples of Tekijuku. (13) *Tekijuku* 1993; (26): 111–55.
16. Matsuki A. *A Short History of Anesthesia in Japan*. p.93–4.
17. Soda H. *An Illustrated History of Medical Culture of Japan*. Kyoto, Shibunkaku Shuppan, 1989. p.320.
18. Matsuki A. *A Short History of Anesthesia in Japan*. p.80.
19. Sato S. Concerning the Effect of Anesthetic Method on the Surgical Operations. *Idan* 1897; (43): 9–12.

Chapter III History of Anesthesia in Japan between 1868 and 1949

1   Otojiro Kitagawa and Spinal Morphine

Since Wang and his associates first reported the use of spinal opioids in human in 1979,[1] and Behar et al described epidural opioid therapy in the same year,[2] these pain control methods have been commonly used worldwide.[3] However, little is known about the fact that the origin of the spinal opioids dates back to the years when the use of spinal anesthesia had just been discovered, and that a Japanese surgeon was one of the pioneers of this method. The discussion in this section focuses on how Otojiro Kitagawa (1864–1922), a surgeon from Nagoya, Japan, came up with the idea of spinal morphine administration.

Otojiro Kitagawa (Figure 3.1.1) was a pioneer in the history of Japanese surgery because he was the first to perform Gasserian ganglion resection for the treatment of intractable trigeminal neuralgia,[4] and he was the first to use morphine for spinal anesthesia in Japan.[5] In an article titled "Nothing New under the sun – a Japanese Pioneer in the clinical use of intrathecal morphine," which appeared in *Anesthesiology* in 1983, I described the Kitagawa's use of morphine for recalcitrant pain.[6] Because the clinical use of spinal morphine was novel in the field of anesthesia at that time, I presented an article titled "Dr. Otojiro Kitagawa, a Japanese pioneer in the clinical use of intrathecal morphine" at the Third International Symposium on the

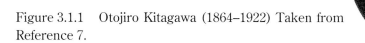

Figure 3.1.1   Otojiro Kitagawa (1864–1922) Taken from Reference 7.

History of Anesthesia in Atlanta in 1992.[7] In this presentation, I stated that Kitagawa was the first to administer spinal morphine to attenuate severe pain because there is no information on the earlier use of this method.

In 2002, 10 years after my presentation, Barros from Chile presented an interesting article at the Fifth International Symposium on the History of Anesthesia held in Santiago, Spain,[8] which claimed that it was not Otojiro Kitagawa but Mathieu Jaboulay (1860–1913) of Lyon, France, who first administered spinal morphine to humans. Barros reported that Dr. Caupolicán Pardo, a Chilean surgeon, visited France to study surgery and authored a paper on spinal anesthesia that was published in *Revista Médica de Chile* in September, 1901.[9] In that report, Pardo mentioned that Jaboulay made a presentation at the Lyon's Society of Surgery on July 15, 1899, wherein he described the use of intrathecal morphine in a patient with intractable cancer pain and achieved a good result.

Although Barros cited Pardo's report to show that Jaboulay was the first to use spinal morphine, Pardo's paper is a secondary source, and no primary source was referenced by Barros. I extensively searched the literature for the primary source on this subject and found that Jaboulay authored no independent paper on the subject, but was able to find an entry alluding to the use of spinal morphine by Jaboulay in the column "Société de Chirurgie de Lyon" in the October 1898 issue of the periodical *Lyon medical*.[10] According to the description, a meeting of the society was held on July 13, 1898 (Pardo incorrectly reported the date as "July 15"), and one of the topics was "Quincke's puncture for trauma in the lumbar region." At the meeting, Jaboulay presented the case of a cancer patient who experienced sharp pain for which he administered cocaine and morphine intrathecally (doses of these agents were not described), and observed pain relief, despite complications such as vertigo and headache. He concluded that this method held therapeutic potential for the treatment of metastatic cancer. Although there was no information on the doses of morphine Jaboulay administered, this is the earliest and most reliable record on the first use of spinal morphine worldwide. Another report on the use of spinal morphine was published the following year,[11] wherein Jaboulay encountered a case of lower limb contracture in a woman with a 1-year history of myelitis. After extracting 5 mL of bloody cerebrospinal fluid, Jaboulay injected 2 mL of a solution (50 mL solution contains 0 gr. 01 centigr. of morphine and 0 gr. 00025 centimilligr. of cocaine) (sic) into the patient's spine. Numbness began in the lower extremities 12 h after injection and subsequently ascended to the level of breasts and then to the rest of the body within 60 h.

The contracted extremities became inert and flexible. The general paralysis lasted for 8 days, during which the patient's bladder and rectum had to be artificially evacuated. Considering the slow onset of analgesia, morphine and cocaine were likely injected into the epidural space.

It should be noted that Jaboulay used morphine with or without cocaine for the control of intractable pain, not for surgical anesthesia. Before this, in June 1897, Jaboulay tried to treat two tetanus patients using spinal injections of anti–tetanus serum; therefore, he must have been familiar with the spinal puncture method.[12]

Although Barros noted that Jaboulay's name appeared on the first page of Kitagawa's paper and concluded that Kitagawa must have known about Jaboulay's work, Barros ignored the other 25 authors appeared in Kitagawa's paper. Nonetheless, most of these 25 authors were not directly associated with the clinical use of spinal morphine before 1900. Unfortunately, Barros overlooked the work of Schiassi, a surgeon from Budrio, Italy, who, in 1900, reported the results of three major operations, a leg amputation, resection of the suprapubic region, and extirpation of a rectal tumor, using spinal anesthesia with cocaine (1 mL of 1% solution). In one of the three operations, he intrathecally injected "0 gr. 003 milligr" (sic) morphine combined with 10 mg of cocaine (1 mL of 1% solution),[13] thus Shiassi used a combined solution of cocaine and morphine for surgical anesthesia.

In his paper, Kitagawa referenced a review article by Hahn (May 1900),[14] in which the use of spinal morphine by Jaboulay and Schiassi was discussed. Considering that Kitagawa referred to the articles by Jaboulay, Schiassi, and Hahn, and that Hahn described the use of spinal morphine by Jaboulay and Schiassi, it appears that Kitagawa obtained the idea for subarachnoid injection of morphine from these papers because Kitagawa used a combined solution of the local anesthetic agent eucaine, instead of cocaine, in combination with morphine for control of intractable pain, rather than surgical anesthesia. Moreover, Marx reported the routine use of cocaine and morphine in a spinal injection to attenuate labor pain in 1900,[15] whereas Matas intrathecally administered the same combination as surgical anesthesia in the same year.[16] Because these authors were not mentioned in Kitagawa's paper, their achievements were excluded from the present discussion.

References and Remarks

1. Wang JK, Nauss LA, and Thomas JE. Pain relief by intrathecally applied

morphine in man. *Anesthesiology* 1979; 50: 149–51.
2. Behar M, Magora F, Olshwang D, and Davidson JT. Epidural morphine in treatment of pain. *Lancet* 1979; 1: 527–9.
3. Ready LB, Oden R, Chadwick HS, Benedetti C, Rooke GA, Caplan R, and Wild LM. Development of an anesthesiology–based postoperative pain management service. *Anesthesiology* 1988; 68: 100–6.
4. Kitagawa O. An intractable trigeminal neuralgia case successfully cured by means of the Gasserian ganglion resection via craniotomy under chloroform anesthesia. *Tokyo Iji Shinshi* 1899; (1123): 1745–51.
5. Kitagawa O. On the spinal anesthesia with cocaine. *Tokyo Iji Shinshi* 1901; (1200): 653–8.
6. Matsuki A. Nothing New under the sun–a Japanese pioneer in the clinical use of intrathecal morphine–. *Anesthesiology* 1983; 58: 289–90.
7. Matsuki A. Dr. Otojiro Kitagawa, A Japanese pioneer in the clinical use of intrathecal morphine. In: Fink BR, Morris LE, and Stephen CR. eds. *Proceeding of The Third International Symposium on the History of Anesthesia*. Park Ridge, Wood Library–Museum of Anesthesiology, 1992. p.288–92.
8. Barros S. Nothing new under the sun – A French (not a Japanese) pioneer in the clinical use of intrathecal morphine. In: Diz JC, Franco A, Bacon DR, Rupreht J, and Alvarez J. eds. *Proceeding of The Fifth International Symposium on the History of Anesthesia*. Amsterdam, Elsevier, 2002. p.189–92.
9. Pardo C. Las Inyecciones Intraraquídeas de Cocaína. *Rev. Med. Chile* 1901; 29: 227–35.
10. Anonym. Société de Chirurgie de Lyon. *Lyon médical* 1898; (41): 196–7.
11. Anonym. Les injections intra–méningées de morphine et de cocaïne comme moyen de traitement des contractures et de l'épilepsie. *La Semaine médicale* 1899; 19: 432.
12. Jaboulay M. Drainage de l'espace sous–arachnoïdien et injection de liquides médicamenteux dans les méninges. *Lyon medical* 1898; (20): 71–2.
13. Schiassi B. Un procédé simplifié de cocaïnization de la moelle. *La Semaine médicale* 1900; 20: 94.
14. Hahn F. Ueber Cocainisierung des Rückenmarkes. Centralblatt für die Grenzgebiete der Medizin und Chirurgie. 1900; 3: 337–41.
15. Marx S. Medullary narcosis during labor. *Medical Record* 1900; 58: 521–7.
16. Matas R. Local and regional anesthesia with cocaine and other analgesic drugs, including the subarachnoid method as applied in general surgical practice. *The Philadelphia Medical Journal* 1900; 6: 820–43.

2 Description of Anesthesia in Japanese Textbooks of General Surgery before 1949

In July 1950, the professor of the First Department of Surgery at Tohoku University School of Medicine, Masao Muto (1898–1972) (Figure 3.2.1) attended Meyer Saklad's informative lectures on anesthesia at the Japanese–American Joint Conference on Medical Education held in Tokyo.[1] Later, Muto wrote a journal entry explaining why he had attended the anesthesia session rather than another session on surgery:

> "When I joined (in 1923) the First Department of Surgery at Tohoku University School of Medicine, which was chaired by Professor Shichitaro Sugimura (1879–1960), general anesthesia had been widely employed, and 4 years as an assistant I had mastered administering general anesthesia. Then, I noticed that spinal and local anesthesia were gaining popularity while general anesthesia had been becoming obsolete since approximately 1930. Because our knowledge of anesthesia is outdated and behind the West by 20 years, I chose to attend the anesthesia session to learn more about the advances in anesthesia practice in the United States."[2]

It was clear from Muto's entry that he recognized there was a trend toward the greater use of local anesthesia including spinal anesthesia, with general anesthesia becoming increasingly obsolete since the 1920s and 1930s. In this section, the aim was to clarify whether this tendency could be traced in the contents of Japanese textbooks of general surgery published before 1949. This was achieved by counting the pages assigned to the descriptions of anesthesia, general anesthesia, and local anesthesia in specific reference texts.

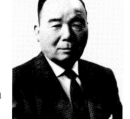

Figure 3.2.1   Masao Muto (1898–1972). Taken from *Tohoku Igaku Zasshi* 1960; 60 (1, 2).

Eighteen popular Japanese textbooks of general surgery were chosen as the materials for this study. Their publication dates ranged from 1880 to 1936: four textbooks from the 1880s, three from the 1890s, four from the 1900s, two from the 1910s, two from the 1920s, and three from 1930s. For each textbook, the total pages were counted together with the number of pages allocated to descriptions of anesthesia, general anesthesia, and local anesthesia. Finally, the ratios of the subsections to the total pages were calculated. Table 3.2.1 summarizes the result.

Table 3.2.1 Description of Anesthesia, General Anesthesia, and Local Anesthesia in 18 Japanese Textbooks of General Surgery published before 1949

Year	Title	Author	Total pages	GA+LA		GA:LA	
			Page		(%)	(%)	(%)
1880	Ermerins' General Surgery[1]	Masazumi Takahashi*	332	0	(0)	0	0
1883	Hueter's General Surgery[2]	Kan Adachi*	1565	0	(0)	0	0
1888	New General Surgery[3]	Masato Toyabe*	676	0	(0)	0	0
1889	General Surgery	Todo Yoshimasu	755	0	(0)	0	0
1890	General Surgery	Eijiro Haga	479	18	(3.8)	89	11
1892	General Surgery[4]	Kaizo Arimatsu*	252	19	(7.5)	95	5
1893	Tillmann's General Surgery[5]	Kanji Uozumi*	1054	47	(4.5)	91	9
1900	Surgery	Shingo Kuroki	304	12	(3.9)	85	15
1906	Concise General Surgery	Taijiro Kawamura	292	23	(7.9)	75	25
1906	New General Surgery	Yosai Shimodaira	1402	52	(3.7)	75	25
1908	Modern General Surgery[6]	Masao Yamamura*	1766	65	(3.7)	78	22
1912	Handy General Surgery	Naozumi Fukushima	466	29	(6.2)	50	50
1913	New Military General Surgery	Futsui Hattori	740	26	(3.5)	26	74
1920	Motegi's General Suregry	Kuranosuke Motegi	635	36	(5.7)	57	43
1928	Japanese General Surgery	Takuma Matsunaga	274	39	(14.2)	61	39
1931	Minor General Surgery	Tetsuzo Aoyama	425	31	(7.3)	63	37
1934	Torikata's General Surgery	Ryuzo Torikata	653	21	(3.2)	50	50
1936	Concise General Surgery	Shigeru Ogawa	579	38	(6.6)	71	29
1955	New General Surgery**	Masao Muto	453	31	(6.8)	70	30

Abbreviations: GA, general anesthesia; LA, local anesthesia; GA+LA, all anesthesia.
1. A transcript of CJ Elmerins' lectures at the Prefectural Osaka Hospital.
2. Hueter C. *Grundriss der Chirurgie*. Leipzig, Vogel, 1880.
3. Agnew DH. *The Principles and Practice of Surgery*. Philadelphia, Lippincott, 1878–83.
4. Original textbook was not identified.
5. Tillmanns H. *Lehrbuch der allgemeinen und speciellen Chirurgie*. Leipzig, Enke, 1892.
6. Lexer E. *Lehrbuch der allgemeinen Chirurgie zum Gebrauche für Arzte und Studenten*. Stuttgart, Enke, 1906.
* translator
** For reference, Muto's textbook of general anesthesia published in 1955 is shown.

No descriptions of local anesthesia were found in any of the four textbooks of general surgery published in the 1880s. Most of them were abridged translations from German textbooks of general surgery or were translations of lectures by a German mentor. This is consistent with the fact that Carl Koller first reported the clinical use of local anesthesia with cocaine in 1884.[3]

In the three textbooks published in the 1890s, anesthesia accounted for an average of 5.2% (range 3.8–7.5%) of pages in the textbooks; however, 91.7% (range 89–95%) of that contents covered the topic of general anesthesia. Thus, general anesthesia appears to have been the focus of education and practice of anesthesia. It is noteworthy that the contents of the anesthesia section produced by Haga (1890) focused on chloroform anesthesia, particularly on the associated complications and their prevention. The contents were as follows:

Anesthetic Method
  General anesthesia
    (a) Hypnotism
    (b) Nitrous oxide (laughing gas)
    (c) Ether
    (d) Chloroform
  I Chloroform anesthesia
    Inhaler of chloroform, conscious stage, excitement stage, and anesthesia stage
    Unpleasant complications of chloroform anesthesia
    Artificial ventilation
    Deaths due to chloroform anesthesia
    Precautions against chloroform inhalation
    Combined anesthesia (morphine and chloroform)
  II Ether anesthesia
Local anesthesia
  Refrigerant anesthesia by ether
  Cocaine: application on the eye, subcutaneous injection, intoxication

The anesthesia contents in the textbook by Arimatsu (1892) were similar, although the description of local anesthesia contained four methods, including compression, refrigeration, skin application (ointment), and subcutaneous injection. In 1892, the Tillmanns' German surgical textbook was published, and a year later, its Japanese translation titled *Chishi Geka Soron* was published. The anesthesia section contained the following contents:

  Analgesic method during operation: general anesthesia, local anesthesia
    Chloroform
      Chloroform anesthesia
      Signs of chloroform anesthesia
      Unpleasant complications of chloroform anesthesia: nausea, respiratory depression, and disturbances in circulatory system
      Occurrence of deaths during chloroform anesthesia and their causes
      Treatment of unpleasant complications during chloroform anesthesia
    Ether anesthesia
    Nitrous oxide anesthesia
    Local anesthesia

With regard to four textbooks of general surgery published in the 1900s, anesthesia was covered by an average of 4.8% of the total number of pages. In addition, the ratio of pages covering general anesthesia to the total pages averaged 78.3% (range 75–85%), which was less than the value of 91.7% in the 1890s. However, the pages assigned to local anesthesia increased from 8.3% in the 1890s to 21.7% in the 1900s, reflecting the growth in local anesthesia in Japan over that time. Scriba was a foreign mentor at the University of Tokyo who was highly influential in Japanese surgery.[4] Because the contents of Kawamura's textbook (Figure 3.2.2) relied on Scriba's lectures, the work unsurprisingly had a significant influence on Japanese surgeons. According to the contents, Scriba believed that spinal, epidural (sacral) anesthesia, and local anesthesia belonged to different categories, perhaps because the concept of "regional anesthesia" had not yet been established by Cushing.[5] Notably, Scriba appeared to advocate the use of chloroform anesthesia, as evidenced by the following contents:

  Anesthetic method
    General anesthesia 1 Nitrous oxide 2 Ether 3 Chloroform
    Chloroform anesthesia
      Properties of chloroform
      Method to identify chloroform
      Inhalation apparatus
      Application of chloroform anesthesia
      Chloroform anesthesia
        1) Conscious stage 2) Excitement stage 3) Anesthesia stage

2   Description of Anesthesia in Japanese Textbooks of General Surgery before 1949   107

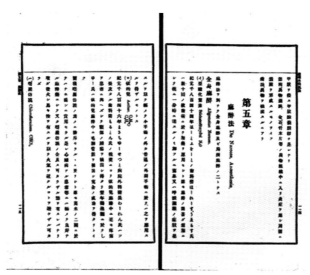

Figure 3.2.2   Title page of Kawamura's *Concise General Surgery* published in 1906.

   Complications during chloroform anesthesia
    1) Vomiting 2) Respiratory abnormalities 3) Disturbed cardiac function
   Deaths due to chloroform anesthesia
  Ether anesthesia
   Inhalation apparatus
  Other anesthetics
  Spinal anesthesia
  Epidural injection method (Sacral anesthesia)
  Local anesthesia
   1) Refrigeration anesthesia 2) Infiltration anesthesia with cocaine

 In the 1910s, 62.0% of the anesthesia pages of the two identified textbooks were devoted to descriptions of local anesthesia, whereas the average number of pages devoted to anesthesia (4.8%) remained unchanged. This was almost three times greater than the 21.7% noted in the preceding period. The marked increase in the coverage of local anesthesia by the 1910s was because of Hattori's textbook *Gunjin Geka Shinron* (*New Military General Surgery*), in which local anesthesia was covered in more than 70% of the pages devoted to anesthesia. This was probably because local anesthesia was

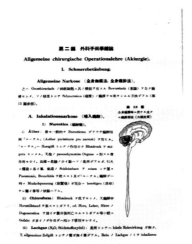

Figure 3.2.3 Title page of *Torikata's General Surgery* published in 1934.

highly recommended for anesthesia in military surgery.

With regard to two textbooks in the 1920s and the three textbooks in the 1930s, the coverage of local anesthesia fell to 41.0% and 38.7%, respectively. Although this coverage was less than it had been in the 1920s, it was still almost twice that in the 1900s. Among the five textbooks in the 1920s and 1930s, local anesthesia was covered to the highest percentage (50%) in the textbook by Torikata (Figure 3.2.3) who preferred it to general anesthesia and denied the use of positive-pressure ventilation in thoracotomy, which seems to reflect his view of anesthesia. The figures from Muto's textbook on general surgery are shown at the bottom of the Table 3.2.1 for reference. The ratio of pages devoted to general and local anesthesia was 7:3, suggesting that more importance was placed on general anesthesia. This may have been because he had enjoyed Saklad's lecture and recognized the importance of general anesthesia featuring tracheal anesthesia.

In total, 18 Japanese textbooks of general surgery published between 1880 and 1949 were reviewed. There was a clear trend for local anesthesia to prevail in Japan from the 1910s, following its development between the 1880s and 1890s in the German-speaking countries. A reason for the high popularity of local anesthesia in Japan in the 1910s was that many Japanese surgeons who played significant roles in the development of the specialty had visited German-speaking countries to study.[6] There was a notable gap of two decades between the trend that observed in the textbooks of general surgery (1910s) and the trend experienced by Muto (1930s) in the 1930s.

References and Remarks

1. Matsuki A. *A Short History of Anesthesia in Japan.* p.161–6.
2. Muto M. A glimpse at advances in anesthetic methods in the United States. *Tohoku Rinsho* 1951; 5: 76–9.
3. Rushman GB, Davies NJH, and Atkinson RS. *A Short History of Anaesthesia –The First 150 Years–.* p.137–40.
4. Reference 1. p.114, p.135.
5. Cushing H. On the avoidance of shock in major amputations by cocainization of large nerve-trunks preliminary to their division. *Ann Surg.* 1902; 36: 321–45.
6. Reference 1. p.113–33.

3   Deaths due to Spinal Anesthesia in Japan before 1945

Spinal anesthesia was first described by August Bier (1861–1949), a professor of surgery at the University of Greifswald, Germany, in 1899.[1] From then, it rapidly spread through Europe and North America,[2,3] and was transmitted to Japan as early as 1900. Independently, the surgeons Kitagawa at Nagoya Koseikan Hospital, Nagoya and Ryohei Azuma (?–?) of Kanazawa Hospital, Kanazawa, each began clinical trials of spinal anesthesia in 1900, and their papers were read in April 1901 at the third Annual Meeting of the Japan Surgical Society (JSS). Kitagawa[4,5] reported six cases of spinal anesthesia, using cocaine during four operations and 10 mg of intrathecal morphine to relieve chronic pain in each of the remaining two patients. Azuma[6] described 29 cases of spinal anesthesia with cocaine for various surgical procedures. Kitagawa became acquainted with the method by means of German and French journals of surgery, whereas Azuma was likely to have obtained his knowledge of the technique from his mentor, Kozo Kimura (1860–1931). Kimura was a professor of surgery at the Medical College of the Fourth High School at Kanazawa;[7] He returned to Japan in December 1899, just 8 months after the publication of Bier's article, and after spending 2 years at the University of Freiburg, Germany. After these two reports, Kawashima and Omi of Professor H. Ito's (1864–1929) Department of Surgery at Kyoto University described 21 surgical operations performed under spinal anesthesia in Japan.[8] Thereafter, the technique was gradually disseminated among surgeons across the country.

As the use of the spinal anesthesia spread across the Western countries, so too did the rate of serious complications from the technique. According to Hahn's review article on spinal anesthesia in April 1901, a score of deaths had been reported just 1.5 years after Bier's original publication.[9] Although not all of them were attributable to spinal anesthesia alone, some of them were clearly associated with the method. Despite the development of hyperbaric solution in 1907 by Baker, a London surgeon, no meaningful efforts were made to avert these complications.[10] The concept of baricity or specific gravity of an anesthetic solution was firmly established in the 1920s and 1930s.[11,12]

Despite a careful review of the medical literature, it is strange that there were no documented deaths due to spinal anesthesia for the first 25 years after its introduction in Japan. This is partially supported by Ueno, who presented a special report on local anesthesia at the 12th Annual Meeting of the JSS in 1911, mentioning that there had been no fatalities associated with spinal anesthesia.[13] It is highly unlikely that this was the case, and there may have been a tendency to neglect reporting deaths due to the procedure. Therefore, further reviews of medical literature could clarify this issue and provide readers with new information on the subject.

In 1926, Chikamori reported sudden respiratory arrest in four patients within several minutes of subarachnoid injection of tropacocaine 50 mg.[14] Two out of four patients recovered spontaneous breathing after artificial ventilation, but the remaining two died soon after the procedure, despite resuscitation. Because the age, exact date of death, and the surgical procedure of each of the latter two patients were not identified, these were not considered the first deaths due to spinal anesthesia in Japan. However, motivated by this tragic experience, Chikamori conducted an animal experiment to investigate the possible factors associated with respiratory arrest.[14] He measured the cerebrospinal fluid (CSF) pressure at the cisternal magna during a spinal injection of tropacocaine, and he observed that this resulted in respiratory depression and a marked decrease in CSF pressure. Consequently, he concluded that a rapid and marked decrease in the CSF pressure was the major causative factor for respiratory arrest leading to death.

In the same year, Obuchi from Keio University Hospital, reported two fatalities due to spinal anesthesia.[15] The first patient, a 30-year-old woman who received spinal anesthesia with 60 mg of tropacocaine for bilateral ovariotomies, developed respiratory arrest and died on April 29, 1925, despite vigorous resuscitation. The second patient, a 45-year-old woman, who received spinal anesthesia with 60 mg of tropacocaine, developed respiratory deterioration that progressed to cardiac arrest. Although spontaneous respiration and heart beats were regained within 1 h of artificial respiration and injections of camphor and lobeline (doses of both drugs unknown), she died 4 days later on April 27, 1925, without recovering consciousness. No autopsies were performed in either case. Obuchi had been using spinal anesthesia since 1918, and these fatal incidents were his first experiences. He concluded that the deaths were related either to the patients' specific constitutions or to cephalad migration of the local anesthetic agents in the subarachnoidal space. These are the first fatalities to be directly associated with spinal anesthesia in Japan; their dates of death, preoperative diagnoses, operations performed, and surgeons were known.

In 1932, Fukamachi and colleagues reported eight fatalities due to spinal anesthesia, which they observed at the Keio University Hospital or affiliated hospitals since 1920.[16,17] The first two patients were the same patients as described in Obuchi's article.[15] The remaining six patients also underwent spinal anesthesia with tropacocaine, although the details of their procedures are unavailable except for one patient who underwent autopsy. This patient was a 32-year-old woman in the tenth month of pregnancy. She had a contracted pelvis and underwent cesarean section under spinal anesthesia using 60 mg of tropacocaine dissolved in 7 ml of her CSF. After injection, she was kept in the supine position; however, she stopped breathing when the skin incision was made (almost simultaneously). The operation was transiently stopped, and artificial ventilation was started, lobeline, a respiratory stimulant, and cardiotonics (name and doses of the latter are unknown) were injected with no discernable effects. The operation was then restarted to deliver the baby, but the patient subsequently died. Unfortunately, the autopsy found no particular pathology and she was therefore diagnosed with status thymicolymphaticus. Although cephalad migration of tropacocaine was most likely to have caused the respiratory arrest, this was excluded from the discussion of the cause of death. At that time, Paltauf's hypothesis of status thymicolymphaticus[18] prevailed among the medical community in Japan.[19] Fukamachi reported the death rate due to spinal anesthesia to be 0.13% or five deaths in 3860 spinal anesthetics, at his institution.[17]

In 1930, Kimura, the chief surgeon of Tokyo Yoikuin, Itabashi, Tokyo, proposed an opposing theory to the central migration of local anesthetic agent as the major cause for respiratory arrest during spinal anesthesia.[20] To confirm his idea, he measured tropacocaine concentrations in the cisternal magna CSF in six patients receiving the lumbar subarachnoid injection of 50–125 mg of 5% tropacocaine. The agent was detected in the CSF in three out of six patients at doses of 0.062 mg to 0.098 mg which was 0.072% to 0.131% of the doses administered. From this observation, Kimura proposed that respiratory depression occurring immediately following spinal anesthesia did not result from the direct effects of local anesthetic agent that had migrated to the cisterna magna.

In the same year, Seo reported a 56-year-old man who died following spinal anesthesia with 1.0 mL of 5% intrathecal tropacocaine for the reposition of a femur fracture.[21] The patient developed unconsciousness, generalized convulsions, and cyanosis when the tourniquet was removed from his leg. Intracardiac injection of adrenaline and cardiac massage were sufficient to regain his cardiac beats, but he died 26 h later. The cardiac arrest was assumed to be due to hypovolemia that was worsened by the loosening of the tourniquet. In the following year, Ishihara described a 33-year-old woman with a Kruckenberg's tumor who received spinal anesthesia with 50 mg of tropacocaine. She also stopped breathing just before the skin incision, and despite the transient effectiveness of artificial ventilation and intracardiac injection of norepinephrine, she died after 8 h.[22]

Three years after Kimura's proposal that respiratory depression was not due to the direct effect of tropacocaine,[20] Shimotsuma and associates conducted a clinical study to access the theory.[23] They described cisternal injections of 0.5–0.6 mL of 5% tropacocaine to ameliorate systemic tonic spasticity in five patients with tetanus. None of them developed pronounced dyspnea or hypotension, although tachypnea, tachycardia, slightly clouded consciousness, and decreased vagal tones were observed in most of them. From these clinical observations, Shimotsuma and his associates surmised that fatal results in spinal anesthesia resulted primarily from systemic hypotension due to the dilated visceral vascular bed, and not from the cephalad movement of local anesthetic agent. The studies by Kimura[20] and Shimotsuma[23] meant that identification of the true cause of respiratory depression was thwarted for a full decade.

In 1935, Mikawa described two fatal cases due to spinal anesthesia with tropacocaine. One patient was a 19-year-old woman who received the removal of an ovarian cyst under spinal anesthesia with tropacocaine 50 mg. Five min after spinal anesthesia and 1 min after the start of operation, the patient became cyanotic and developed cardiac arrest. Despite vigorous resuscitation, she died four days later without recovering consciousness. The other patient was a 37-year-old woman who also received an ovarian cyst removal under spinal anesthesia with tropacocaine 50 mg. 20 min after spinal injection she became cyanotic and bradycardia was recognized, which was followed by tonic and clonic convulsions and died next day without regaining consciousness. Although Mikawa concluded that the first patient died due to idiosyncrasy (no autopsy was performed) because the patient's father died suddenly during surgery with details remained unknown, and that the second patient died metabolic alkalosis. His conclusions were misleading, and the patients must have been died primarily due to severe respiratory depression caused by cephalad migration of tropacocaine.[24]

In the period between 1933 and 1941, 21 fatalities from spinal anesthesia were reported in medical journals. This number probably only represents the tip of the iceberg. Although various factors were proposed at that time to explain the fatalities associated with spinal anesthesia, no effective or definite measures were suggested to prevent or manage the respiratory depression.[25]

In 1940, Professor Makoto Saito (1889–1950) and Park of Nagoya University described a safer spinal anesthesia technique that involved regulating the level of anesthesia with a hyperbaric solution. Interestingly, it appears that a personal experience may have led Saito to develop this new spinal anesthesia technique. In the autumn of 1937, Saito received spinal anesthesia with a hypobaric solution for appendectomy. Partly because of the need for multiple lumbar punctures, the level of anesthesia ascended to the cervical dermatomes, resulting in him developing dyspnea and dysphonia. Fortunately, Saito spontaneously recovered from this complication without any resuscitative measures or drugs. Thus, Saito was driven by a serious concern about the safety of spinal anesthesia and asked Park, who joined the department in the previous year, to help him devise a safer technique. After strenuous and ingenious experimentation over 2 years, Park perfected a new technique of hyperbaric spinal anesthesia using dibucaine in a 10% glucose solution, and successfully applied it to various surgeries. This new method provided control over the ascent of the level of anesthesia by using a hyperbaric solution in combination with a tilted operating table. He read a paper on this new method at the 41st Annual Meeting of the JSS in 1940,[26] and his paper subsequently appeared in the society's journal.[27] Saito was assiduous in popularizing the newly devised method; however, it did not gain traction as rapidly as he had intended because the Pacific War broke out just 4 months after publication.

In October 1942, in the midst of the Pacific War, Saito hosted the Sixth Annual Meeting of the Japan Surgical Association at Nagoya and presided over a round-table discussion "On Spinal Anesthesia." Saito and seven participants discussed incidents related to the method. At the beginning of the discussion, he argued that spinal anesthesia would be more important than ever before and would be used much more frequently because medical and pharmaceutical products were in short supply due to the wartime effort. Yoichi Azuma (1897–?), a professor of the Second Department of Surgery at Kumamoto Medical College, Kumamoto, made a striking comment on the subject, as follows:

> You, who are participating in this discussion, may have experienced accidents with spinal anesthesia. You may know several potential causes for troubles in which respiratory deterioration leads to death; of course, it is more likely that the respiratory center in the medulla oblongata will be paralyzed in such cases. Although I don't want to tell you who did it or where it was done, some investigators conducted an experiment with

spinal anesthesia on convicts under sentence of death. Several convicts were given incremental doses of dibucaine, a local anesthetic, by cisternal puncture until they died. A given dose of the agent caused death in one subject, but not in others, and a marked individual difference was observed in doses of the agent needed to induce death. Consequently, it is likely that cephalad migration of the drug might cause paralysis of the respiratory center in accidents due to spinal anesthesia. However, because there was a marked individual difference in the doses needed to cause paralysis of the respiratory center, it is impossible to predict beforehand who would be sensitive to the agent and who would not.[28]

No questions were asked after Azuma's talk. Although I failed to identify the investigators that had conducted this human experimentation or even the location and date the experiment was performed, it is the only known case of human experimentation in the medical history of Japan to use convicts sentenced to death. According to Azuma's remark, it is apparent that the concept of individual differences in dose requirements or in the dose–response relationship did not pervade anesthetic theory among Japanese surgeons at that time.

In the period between 1942 and 1945, nine fatalities were reported due to spinal anesthesia.[29] Shishito of the First Department of Surgery, Tohoku University reported a death rate of 0.34% (4 deaths out of 1163 spinal anesthetics).[30] In reality, many more fatalities were likely to have occurred, but were unlikely to be reported because of the ongoing war. Moreover, if reported, such accidents would have gained little attention in the medical community at that time.

As mentioned, the number of deaths reported due to spinal anesthesia must have been the tip of the iceberg, probably accounting for less than 10% of the total cases. Extrapolating from these statistics, at least 400–600 patients would have died between 1901 and 1945 as a direct consequence of the method.[31] However, no lawsuits were instituted because the deaths were primarily considered due to the impurity of local anesthetics used or individual thymicolymphatic diatheses, regardless of the results of postmortem dissection. It was unfortunate that an even less desirable situation awaited the Japanese medical community in the decades after the war, because military surgeons with inadequate training for spinal anesthesia returned to practice the method.

References and Remarks

1. Bier A. Versuch über Cocainisirung des Rückenmarkes. *Deutsch Z. Chir.* 1899; 51: 361–9.
2. Rushman GB, Davies NJH, and Atkinson RS. *A Short History of Anaesthesia –The First 150 Years–*. Oxford, Butterworth Heinemann, 1996. p.144–8.
3. Larson MD. History of Anesthetic Practice. In: Miller RD. ed. *Miller's Anesthesia*. (7th ed.) Philadelphia, Churchill Livingstone, 2010. p.21–2.
4. Kitagawa O. On spinal anesthesia with cocaine. *J. Japan Surgical Society* 1901; 3: 185–91.
5. Matsuki A. Dr. Otojiro Kitagawa, A Japanese Pioneer in the Clinical Use of Intrathecal Morphine. In: Fink BR, Morris LE, and Stephen CR. eds. *The History of Anesthesia The Third International Symposium*. Park Ridge, Wood Library–Museum of Anesthesiology, 1992. p.288–92.
6. Azuma R. On duralinfusion. *J. Japan Surgical Society* 1901; 3: 192–7.
7. Kanazawa Medical School was merged into The fourth High School at Kanazawa, and its hospital was called as Kanazawa Hospital at that time. The school developed to become the present Kanazawa University Graduate School of Medicine.
8. Kawashima H, and Omi K. Experiments on Bier's spinal anesthesia with cocaine. *Tokyo Igakukai Zasshi* 1901; 15(17): 1–53.
9. Hahn F. Ueber subarachnoideale Cocaininjectionen nach Bier. *Central Grenz Med. Chir.* 1901; 4: 305–17, 340–54.
10. Barker A. Clinical experiences with spinal analgesia in 100 cases and some reflections on the procedure. *British Medical Journal* 1907; 1: 665–74.
11. Pitkin GP. Controllable spinal anesthesia. *Am J Surg* 1928; 5: 537–53.
12. Sise LF. Pontocaine–Glucose Solution for Spinal Anesthesia. *Surgical Clinics North America* 1935; 15: 1501–11.
13. Ueno N. On local anesthesia. *J. Japan Surgical Society* 1911; 12: 129–62.
14. Chikamori M. New discussions on the cause of death due to lumbar spinal anesthesia. *Chosen Igaku Zasshi* 1926; 69; 921–4.
15. Ohbuchi M. Recent experience of two fatal cases of spinal anesthesia. *Rinsho Sanka Fujinka* 1926; 1: 33–8.
16. Fukamachi A, Amamiya H, and Tonohara K. An autopsy case of spinal death. *Nihon Fujinkagakkai Zasshi* 1930; 5: 87.
17. Fukamachi A, Amamiya H, and Tonohara K. An autopsy case of spinal death. – appendix: pro and con of the use of spinal anesthesia in the terminal stage of pregnancy–. *Rinsho Sanka Fujinka* 1932; 7: 125–35.
18. Paltauf A. Über die Beziehungen der Thymus zum Plötzlichen Tod. *Wiener klinische Wochenschrift* 1889; 2: 877–81.
19. Matsuki A. *The Origin of Anesthesiology, continued*. Tokyo, Shinkokoeki Ishoshuppanbu, 2009. p.132–52.
20. Kimura T. An application of lumbar spinal anesthesia for upper abdominal anesthesia. *J. Japan Surgical Society* 1930; 31: 1330.

21. Seo S. An acute cardiac arrest due to spinal anesthesia and intracardiac injection of adrenalin. *Rinsho Igaku* 1930; 18: 65–77.
22. Ishihara S. Concerning respiratory arrest by spinal anesthesia. *Chiryo to Shoho* 1931; 12: 739–41.
23. Shimotsuma K, Imakawa T, and Han G. Clinical doubt on respiratory paralysis theory in spinal anesthesia with tropacocaine. *Manshu Igaku Zasshi* 1933;19: 463–76.
24. Mikawa M. Two fatal cases due to spinal anesthesia with tropacocain. *Kinki Fijinka Gakkai Zasshi* 1935; 18: 833–46.
25. Matsuki A. *Deaths Associated with Spinal Anesthesia. (Revised ed.)* Tokyo, Kokuseido Shuppan, 2001. p.82.
26. Park RS. Controlled spinal anesthesia by means of an application of hyperbaricity. *J. Japan Surgical Society* 1940; 41: 678–82.
27. Park RS. Controlled spinal anesthesia using hyperbaric local anesthetic solution. *J. Japan Surgical Society* 1941; 42: 805–64.
28. Saito M, Azuma Y, Imazu K, Shimada N, Shirabe R, Tashiro K, Sakakibara T. and Park RS. Round Table discussion "Spinal Anesthesia." *Nihon Rinsho Gekaikai Zasshi* 1943; 7: 113–22.
29. Reference 25. p.82–3.
30. Shishito S, and Mekawa H. Spinal anesthesia–on its side effects–. *J. Japan Surgical Society*. 1944; 45: 5–6.
31. There are no reliable statistics regarding the number of spinal anesthesia administered annually before 1945. Assuming a frequency of 30,000 patients receiving spinal anesthesia each year and a death rate of 0.13% (by Fukamachi[16]), the fatalities would have been 39 each year.

4 The Blank 20 Years in the History of Anesthesia between 1925 and 1945 -The Lost 20 Years-

A notorious debate on the thoracotomy method between Professor Ryuzo Torikata(1878–1952) (Figure 3.4.1) of Kyoto University and Professor Shigeki Sekiguchi(1880–1942) (Figure 3.4.2) of Tohoku University was considered one of the most causative factors that hampered the development of modern anesthesia practice in Japan before the end of the Pacific War in 1945. The debate began at the 26th Annual Meeting of the JSS in 1925 and lasted until the 39th Annual Meeting of the JSS in 1938, at which Torikata was the president at the meeting.[1] It was unfortunate that Japanese surgeons overlooked the remarkable advances in the United States and United Kingdom during the 1920s and 1930s, which would form the basis of modern anesthesiology. Among these, the introduction of a new intravenous anesthetic agent (thiopental), the development of a new tracheal intubation technique, a carbon oxide absorber devise, and the re-introduction of a hyperbaric solution in spinal anesthesia.[2]

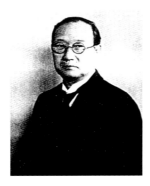

Figure 3.4.1 Ryuzo Torikata (1878–1952). Taken from *Collected Papers and Abstracts from Torikata's Department of Surgery*, Special issue for Torikata's Sixty Anniversary, published in 1941.

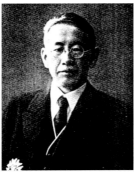

Figure 3.4.2 Shigeki Sekiguchi (1880–1942). Taken from *Collected Papers for Professor Sekiguchi's Sixty Anniversary. Special Issue of J. of Tohoku Meidical Society*, Volume 28, 1941.

Since 1870, when the Meiji Government adopted the German style of medical education, research, and care as a model, surgeons and physicians of other specialties in Japan considered German medicine as the best in the world and American and British medicine as second best.[3] Consequently, The Japanese surgeons overlooked progresses made in the United States and United Kingdom, particularly in the specialty of anesthesia, which was not considered important in its own right , but was instead to be a supplement to surgery. In this context, it is perhaps unsurprising that no Japanese surgeon fully appreciated the importance of advances in anesthesia at that time because they were viewed as part of pointless supplement of second-rate American and British surgery. Shinobu Miyamoto (1911–1987), a professor of surgery at Nihon University School of Medicine, performed thoracotomy according to Torikata's method (i.e., without using positive-pressure ventilation) for pulmonary tuberculosis before 1950. He described the dark side of the debate as follows:

> Because the safety of thoracotomy without positive-pressure ventilation was overly emphasized, and postoperative complications after general anesthesia were feared, the use of anesthesia with positive-pressure ventilation was denounced. Subsequently, it deserves a special attention that tracheal anesthesia was not introduced from the United States to Japan before the outbreak of the Pacific War. On this point, the dark side of the debate is distinctly exposed.[4]

Fujita, a practitioner of anesthesia in Kyoto who was interested in the history of the specialty, was the first anesthesiologist to criticize the debate from the viewpoint of the specialty. One of his conclusions was as follows:

> The debate from the middle of the 1920s to the beginning of the 1930s should have been focused on how safely the chest was opened and how reliable surgical procedures were possible. However, surgeons made no efforts to achieve these goals by dedicated research to establish the theory and practice of modern anesthetic management using an anesthetic apparatus. Thoracic surgeries were instead performed under local anesthesia with incremental doses of morphine and scopolamine based on Torikata's opinion that lateral thoracotomy of the chest, and even bilateral thoracotomy, could be performed safely without positive-pressure ventilation. Thus, only limited thoracic procedures could be performed.[5]

Fujita indicated another important conclusion, as follows:

> Safe and reliable anesthesia was indispensable for smooth and uncomplicated thoracic procedures, however, in Japan, this important anesthetic practice was in the hands of neophyte surgeons in university hospitals. Although this fact should not be neglected, it has not been discussed by surgeons before.[5]

Thus, there was a traditional education system in surgical departments in Japan, in which the practice of anesthesia was considered an appendix to the main practice of surgery. Unfortunately, this denied young surgeons the opportunities to develop specific interest in anesthesia and to develop safer methods of anesthesia. Inamoto, one of Torikata's disciples who later became a professor of anesthesiology at Kyoto University, presented his paper on the debate in 1994 at the symposium of the Japan Society for Clinical Anesthesia. He concluded that the debate had become ridiculous when considering that anesthesiologists later began to practice positive–pressure ventilation under tracheal anesthesia with an anesthetic apparatus.[6] To understand the debate, it is necessary to appreciate the yearly changes in Torikata's opinion of thoracotomy. At the beginning of the debate in 1925, Torikata described his opinion as follows:

> Anyway, we have to accumulate many basic findings to decide whether patients who are able to undergo a thoracotomy without positive–pressure ventilation apparatus are exceptional or patients who are unable to undergo it without the apparatus are exceptional.[7]

In 1926, the following year, Torikata's opinion had evolved, as follows:

> A positive–pressure ventilation apparatus is absolutely unnecessary in our animal experiments and clinical experience. We insist that no adverse finding is observed, even if the chest is opened unilaterally, provided that the duration of the procedure is no more than one and a half hours without applying positive–pressure ventilation. This is a firmly established fact and there is no need for further discussion.[8]

Torikata continued to study the topic and his final aim was being to disseminate his preferred method of thoracotomy among surgeons throughout Japan. For this purpose, he asserted that he wanted to drive any positive–pressure ventilation apparatus out from the JSS.[9] In 1938, at the 39th Annual Meeting of the JSS, at which Torikata was the president, he made rigorous comments as a member of the JSS, not as the president, in a discussion with Professor Shichiro Goto from Kyushu University. Torikata's comments were as follow:

> Our opinion is quite different from that of French surgeons. Their opinion is that positive–pressure ventilation is reasonable, but they perform thoracotomy without the apparatus because it is cumbersome to use. Our opinion is that such an apparatus is injurious, and that we should refrain from using such a harmful apparatus.[9]

> It is quite inadequate only to say that thoracotomy without the apparatus is better than that with it. We are strongly insisting that such an apparatus should not be used to avoid postoperative complications.[10]

As mentioned before, Torikata initially insisted that the chest "could" be opened safely without any support of positive–pressure ventilation; however, his opinion evolved to an extreme view that positive–pressure ventilation was "injurious" during thoracotomy because it caused untoward pulmonary complications. Worse still, because Torikata was so influential at the JSS, both senior and young Japanese surgeons inevitably followed his opinion, and neglected modern anesthetic techniques that were being rapidly devised in the United States.

As described in Slide 42, Chapter I, another significant factor that impeded the progress of anesthesia in Japan before 1945 was the paper presented by Taniguchi in 1924 at the 25th Annual Meeting of the JSS. He came from the First Department of Surgery at Kyushu University, presided by Professor Hayami Miyake (1867–1945). Taniguchi reported that the postoperative mortality rates within 1 month of surgery, for patients undergoing gastric procedures, dramatically improved after using local anesthesia instead of general anesthesia, as shown below:

General anesthesia group
   November 1904–April 1914   33.1% (58 deaths in 177 patients)
   May 1914–December 1919   29.3% (52 deaths in 179 patients)
Local anesthesia group
   January 1920–December 1923   16.3% (30 deaths in 186 patients)

January 1924–December 1927   12.4% (26 deaths in 209 patients)
      (The figures for 1924–1927 were not included in Taniguchi's original presentation and cited for reference from Kuru's review article.[11])

Surgeons are most concerned about the fatal complications in the intraoperative and postoperative periods. Consequently, it was natural that many surgeons hesitated to use general anesthesia and preferred local anesthesia. In addition, they would be less likely to conduct research on general anesthesia. One can be left in no doubt of the serious situation of Japanese surgery at the time, which was dominated not only by Torikata's dogmatic opinion of thoracotomy, but also by grave yet academic figures, of the mortality rate in patients undergoing gastric surgery in Miyake's department. Together, these were the most significant obstacles to the advancement of anesthesia between 1925 and 1945. We can consider these the lost 20 years in the development of anesthesia in Japan.

References and Remarks

1. Anonym. The 39th Annual Meeting of the JSS. *J. Japan Surgical Society* 2000; 101: S113, S146–9.
2. Keys TE. *The History of Surgical Anesthesia*. New York, Schuman's, 1945. p.114–7.
3. Matsuki A. *A Short History of Anesthesia in Japan*. p.111–5.
4. Miyamoto S. *My History of Surgery in the Showa Era*. Tokyo, Nihon Hyoronsha, 1985. p.146.
5. Fujita T. The history of developments of anesthesia for thoracic surgery in the Meiji, Taisho, and Showa eras. (2) – reviewing the controversy on thoracotomy with or without positive–pressure ventilation – . *Rinsho Masui* 1994; 18: 589–91.
6. Inamoto A. Learning from the history of a medical controversy in Japan, concerning thoracotomy with or without positive–pressure ventilation. *J. Japan Society for Clinical Anesthesia* 1994; 14: 216–8.
7. Aoyagi Y. ed. *Collected Papers and Abstracts from Torikata's Department of Surgery*. Kyoto, Geka Hokan Editorial Board, 1941. p.400.
8. ibid. p.404.
9. ibid. p.440.
10. ibid. p.443.
11. Kuru M. Advances in surgery. *J. Japan Medical Association* 1953; 29: 299–319.

5 Hayao Nakatani, Another Surgeon who Appreciated Modern American Anesthesiology in the 1930s

Japanese surgeons and physicians considered German surgery and medicine as the best in the world. This idea had been handed down from their predecessors since the beginning of the Meiji era, when in 1870 Japan had adopted the German model. This is supported by the fact that no topics raised by advances in American surgery were discussed in the round–table talk in 1931, titled "Reminiscences of Japanese Surgery."[1] Furthermore, Tsugushige Kondo (1866–1944), emeritus professor of surgery at the First Department of the University of Tokyo, recalled his memories of surgery at a round–table discussion in 1936, and did not refer to American surgery.[2] In addition, at the round–table talk held in 1960 in remembrance of Professor Tetsuzo Aoyama (1882–1953; the successor of Kondo at the First Department of Surgery of the University of Tokyo), Wakabayashi,[3] a professor of surgery at Nihon University, commented that Professor Aoyama had not appreciated American surgery as superior to German surgery. These reports are further supported by the fact that only one American anesthetic machines was imported to Japan before 1945 by surgeons.

Although American surgery was considered second–rate by most Japanese surgeons at that time, some surgeons did visit medical schools, institutions, and hospitals in the United States. This was mostly on their way to or from Germany and other European countries, and because their main aim was to observe American surgical procedures, most neglected to observe the practice of American anesthesia. However, there are always exceptions to the rule. In the 1930s, three exceptional Japanese surgeons visited hospitals in the United States and wrote papers evaluating American anesthesiology as being excellent, advocating its introduction to Japan. Daisuke Nagae and Kenji Tanaka were among these surgeons, as mentioned in slides 45–55 of Chapter Ⅰ. The other surgeon, and the focus of this section is Hayao Nakatani (1902–1992) (Figure 3.5.1) who was from the First Department of Surgery at the University of Tokyo.

Hayao Nakatani graduated from the University of Tokyo in 1926 and joined the First Department of Surgery of the university run by Professor Aoyama. After receiving his Ph.D from the university in 1933,[4] he worked for the Imperial Women's College of Medicine, Nagasaki Medical College, and other institutions before the end of the Pacific War. After the war, he was a professor of surgery at Toho College of Medicine and then the chief

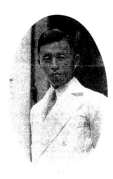

Figure 3.5.1 Hayao Nakatani (1902–1992). With kind permission from the library of Nagasaki University School of Medicine.

of surgery at Tokyo Teishin Hospital. He finally became the director of a branch of Den–en Chofu Central Hospital in Tokyo.

In June 1933, after visiting Germany and the United States, he described a paper titled "Current status of anesthesia in Europe and the United States"[5] in which he introduced the anesthetic practices of these countries. The paper is considered significant to the history of anesthesia in Japan because he advocated that American practices of anesthesia be introduced in Japanese surgery. Although most Japanese surgeons at that time ignored it. He describes the following:

> In a period between June 1932 and April 1933, I visited several teaching hospitals in Europe and the United States. Having observed recent advances in surgery in these countries, I realized that the progress in anesthesia has enormously contributed to that of surgery. This trend is most pronounced in the United States. I therefore wrote this paper to reconsider the status of the current practice of anesthesia in our country, where less attention has been paid to this issue. I would like to ask readers to carefully read and criticize the paper.[5]

In June 1932, Nakatani visited the University of Tübingen, Germany, because Professor Aoyama advised him to do so. He stayed there for 6 months, where he observed surgical operations performed by Professor Martin Kirshner (1879–1936), who had devised a new method of spinal anesthesia that used hypobaric solution by a high pressure method. (Figure 3.5.2). Then, Nakatani moved to Berlin, where he observed surgical procedures by Professor Ferdinand Sauerbruch (1875–1951) at Charité Hospital, where Max Tiegel's anesthetic apparatuses were frequently used for general anesthesia. Moving to Munich and Leipzig, Nakatani learned

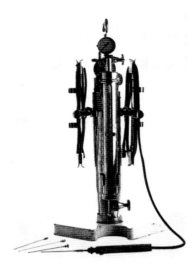

Figure 3.5.2 Kirschner's instrument for high pressure local anesthesia. Taken from Schulte am Esch J and Goerig M. eds. *Catalogue of the exhibition at the Museum für Kunst und Gewerbe, Humburg*, published in 1997.

the technique of flexible gastroscopy from Dr. Schindler and Dr. Henning, respectively. The technique of using a flexible gastroscope was quite new to him and had not yet been introduced in Japan. Thereafter, he visited Vienna and Paris where he did not obtain any useful information. In Germany, he was concerned with the new local anesthetic "spinocaine," Kirschner's new method of spinal anesthesia, a newly developed intravenous agent "evipan sodium," and new anesthetic apparatuses (Franken type from Freiburg and Tiegel type from Berlin). However, he seemed unimpressed by these advancements. He sailed across the Atlantic to the United States via London in March 1933.

In the United States, he visited several hospitals, but mainly stayed at the Mayo Clinic for several weeks. In the clinic, he found the existence of physician anesthetists and nurse anesthetists to be quite novel to him. He mentioned that medical schools in Detroit, Cleveland, and Ann Arbor offered specific training in anesthesia that would be indispensable for the advance in surgery in the future. He was impressed by the elegant induction of anesthesia by anesthesia specialists and that they could respond to any physiological changes in surgical patients during surgery and could use the inhalation of carbon dioxide at the end of a surgical procedure. Surgeons could therefore concentrate their attention on the procedure at hand, while anesthetists focused on the anesthetic management of their patients. Such teamwork between the surgeons and the anesthetists was an enviable proposition to him because he had not observed it in Europe.

He wrote that there were three varieties of anesthetic machines used in the United States, namely the Foregger type (from New York), the McKesson type (from Chicago), and the Lundy–Heidbrink type (from the Mayo Clinic). Cylinders of ethylene, carbon dioxide, nitrous oxide, and oxygen were equipped to these machines. He continued to describe that special attention was paid to prevent explosive and other accidents. Among the gases, nitrous oxide was most frequently used with or without ether. Ethylene was also administered with oxygen through a naso–tracheal tube. Current anesthetic machines were also equipped with a canister that contained calcium oxide and sodium hydroxide to economize on the gases by reusing them after absorbing carbon dioxide. By using these canisters, the consumption of gases decreased to less than 25% of the previous levels.

Although the main purpose of tracheal intubation is to secure the airway, Nakatani described it as a means of preventing ethylene from leaking in the operating room. In 1933, when Nakatani stayed at the Mayo Clinic, 708 patients were administered general anesthesia using tracheal intubation, of which 405 were for head and neck surgery. When compared with approximately 100 surgical procedures per day in total, three cases on an average day for which naso–tracheal anesthesia was performed was a small number. Therefore, he was unlikely to fully recognize the significance of naso–tracheal intubation in the practice of anesthesia. If he had appreciated it more and described the practice of tracheal intubation in detail, he may have made a stronger impact on Japanese surgeons and the subsequent progress in the specialty. In his conclusion, Nakatani made the following statement:

> I briefly described the status of anesthesia practice in Europe and the United States. In short, it is apparent that anesthesia is a part of surgical practice and is significantly associated with patient's prognosis. Consequently, we should not only be satisfied with local anesthesia using procaine, spinal anesthesia using tropacocaine, and the open drop method using ether, but we should also pay more attention to recent advances in anesthesia. Anesthesia with nitrous oxide has little effect on arterial blood pressure or the parenchymal organs, and it is excreted rapidly, thereby decreasing the chance of shock. It would be ideal to make wide use of nitrous oxide, if it is financially possible for clinical use in Japan.

Given this description, it is clear that Nakatani correctly evaluated the

American practice of anesthesia and understood anesthesia to be a key to the future advancement of surgery. He observed that the current practice of anesthesia in the United States was more advanced than that in Germany. This was evidenced by several factors, including the existence of specialists and an educational system for their training; the variety of anesthetic machines available; the use of a rebreathing system with a carbon oxide absorber; the advance in naso–tracheal intubation; and the existence of a piping system in the operating room. His understanding of anesthesia was consistent with the subsequent history of the specialty.

Unfortunately, there is no evidence that the practice of anesthesia in Japan improved after Nakatani's article. Because the academic regime of the JSS was dominated by the influence of German surgery, one can understand why a brief article by a young and spirited surgeon that strongly advocated the American system of anesthesiology did not attract any attention.

One final point regarding the possible relationship between Nakatani and Nagae is worth noting. Nakatani graduated from the University of Tokyo in 1926, and Nagae graduated from the same university in 1929. Both joined the First Department of Surgery run by Professor Aoyama. Nagae completed his Ph.D research in 1934–1935, was still working when Nakatani returned home from the visits to Germany and the United States in April 1933.

After returning, one can only assume that Nakatani discussed his experience of German and American surgery at the departmental conference, and that Nagae may have been present in the audience. It is therefore plausible that Nagae was impressed by Nakatani's talk, featuring the importance of anesthesia and the high standard of the subject in the United States, particularly at the Mayo Clinic and may have become determined to visit the Mayo Clinic visiting the United States as a medical attaché at the Japanese Embassy in Washington D.C. 3 years later. Nagae's case is an extremely exceptional one in the history of anesthesia in Japan because there is no surgeon in the period between 1868 and 1945 who studied anesthesia in a foreign country for more than 6 months.

In 1983, some 50 years after his study abroad, Nakatani wrote an essay titled "Abroad fifty years ago"[6] in which he stated:

> The United States is now at the leading edge of the specialty of surgery; however, the United States was perceived to be behind Germany at that time. It was disappointing that because of the Pacific War, the United States opened a huge gap in surgical practice over our country.[6]

The single largest cause for this huge gap between the two countries was that Japanese surgeons overlooked the rapidly advancing American practice of anesthesia, despite it being mentioned repeatedly.

References and Remarks

1. Miwa Y, Shiota H, Kimura K, Sato S, Haga E, Hayashi H, Tashiro Y, Okada W, Kondo T, Fujimaki K, Oda H, and Matsumoto F. (presided by Motegi K.) Reminiscences of Japanese Surgery. *J. Japan Surgical Society* 1931; 32: 431–43.
2. Kondo T, Ikeda T, Kuzuhara T, Sassa R, Hirose W, and Sakai T. Listening to Emeritus Professor Kondo's Recollections of Surgery. *Rinsho no Nihon*. 1936; 4: 68–87.
3. Alumni Association of the First Department of Surgery at the University of Tokyo. ed. *Essays in celebration of the 100th Anniversary of Professor Tetsuzo Aoyama's Birth. The History of the First Department of Surgery at the University of Tokyo.* (2nd issue) Tokyo, The First Department of Surgery at the University of Tokyo, 1960. p.124.
4. Nakatani's thesis for Ph.D. was as given below.
   Nakatani H. Experimentelle Untersuchungen über den Einfliss des Blutes auf die örtliche pyrogene Infektion. *Arch. klin Chir*. 1932; 170: 648–71.
5. Nakatani H. Current status of anesthesia in Europe and the United States. *Iji Koron* 1933; (1992): 4, (1993): 4–5.
6. Reference 2. p.80–2.

6 Professor Saito, Dr. Park, and Terminal Sac Anesthesia
–The First to Propose the Designation of *Saddle Block* Technique in the World–

In his monograph published in 1955, Parmley[1] described that, in 1946, Adriani was the first to develop the special regional block to anesthetize the perineal region and to coin the term "saddle block" technique. This is evidenced by the fact that Adriani did not use this phrase in his 1945 article on spinal anesthesia[2] and that no mention was made on the subject in the 1942 edition of Lundy's textbook of anesthesia.[3] Although Lundy used the phrase "low spinal anesthesia" for the same technique proposed by Adriani, he neither made a clear definition of the technique nor employed a specific designation. The opinion that Adriani was the first to propose the saddle block technique was also accepted by Fink,[4] and by Jacob and colleagues.[5] However, it is unknown, even to many Japanese anesthesiologists and medical historians, that the same technique had already been performed clinically as early as 1940 in Japan, which precedes the description of Adriani by 6 years. Professor Saito's episode, which led him to develop a safer method of spinal anesthesia, was briefly described in slides 23–25 of Chapter I and the second section of this chapter.

As mentioned, Saito fortunately survived respiratory depression due to ascent of the level of spinal anesthesia while using a hypobaric solution. This incident motivated him to devise a safer technique of spinal anesthesia. He therefore asked Park Rang-Su (1908–1945) (Figure 3.6.1), a junior member of the department, to investigate the subject and develop a new method. After repeated experiments using a glass model of the human spinal column (Figure 3.6.2), Park studied the movement of local anesthetic agent

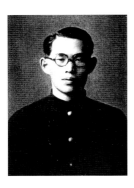

Figure 3.6.1   Park Rang-Su (1908–1945). Taken from Matsuki A. *Professor Saito and Spinal Anesthesia*, published in 2000.

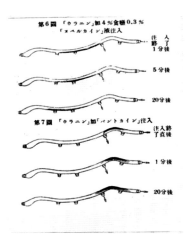

Figure 3.6.2　Glass model of human spinal column. Taken from Reference 6.

colored by dye (fluorescein sodium) in the model column, and found that a hyperbaric solution with 10% glucose solution was useful to control the extent of spread of the local anesthetic solution when the operating table was also tilted. By April 1939, he had eventually perfected a safer technique that used the new hyperbaric solution and had successfully applied it in various surgical operations. During the year from April 1939 to March 1940, Park and associates administered the new method to approximately 370 patients, with just one fatality during that time. Importantly, this death was due to purulent peritonitis and was not directly attributable to the anesthetic method. Park[6] read his paper on the subject at the 41th Annual Meeting of the JSS in April 1940, and his paper[7] appeared in the August issue of the Journal of the JSS in 1941 with additional patient data. The number of patients given spinal anesthesia had increased from 370 to 464 by June 1940 when the paper was submitted to the journal for publication.

Among the 464 patients, Park gave *intradurale Sacralanästhesie* (intradural sacral anesthesia) to 72 patients who underwent hemorrhoidectomy, anal fistulectomy, incision of perianal abscess, or cystoscopy. His definition of *Intradurale Sacralanästhesie* is as follows:

In this method, sacral nerve paralysis is only produced because a hyperbaric local anesthetic solution injected in the subarachnoid space gravitates to the sacral sac. Therefore, the method can be called *intradurale Sacralanästhesie* as opposed to the *sacral anesthesia* or *sacral epidural anesthesia*.[8]

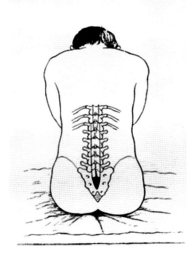

Figure 3.6.3　Sitting position after intrathecal injection. Taken from Reference 6.

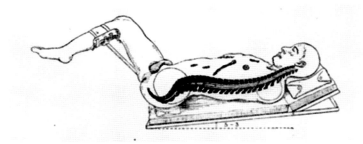

Figure 3.6.4　Patient position in perineal surgery. Taken from Reference 6.

His method of *"intradurale Sacralanästhesie"* and the patient's position are described as follows:

> With the patient in a sitting position, 1.0 mL of a hyperbaric solution of local anesthetic is injected intrathecally through the intervertebral space between the fourth and fifth lumbar vertebrae. The patient is kept in the sitting position for several minutes to allow the agent to descend into the sacral sac. (Figures 3.6.3 and 3.6.4)[8]

It is apparent that Park clearly defined the "saddle block" method and used it with his patients. Later, Professor Saito revised the term *intradurale*

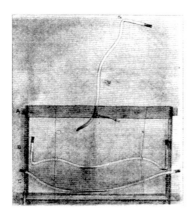 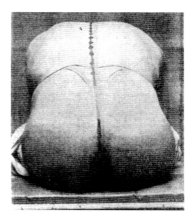

Figure 3.6.5 Glass model of human spinal column. Taken from Reference 11.

Figure 3.6.6 Sitting position for saddle block. Taken from Reference 11.

Sacralanästhesie to *terminal sac anesthesia*[9] or *spinal terminal sac anesthesia*[10] to avoid confusion because *intradurale Sacralanästhesie* could imply *sacral plexus block* or *caudal anesthesia*.

Despite the evidence, Barker, a surgeon from London, must be considered the first to describe the concept of hyperbaricity in the practice of spinal anesthesia.[11-13] He demonstrated the migration of an anesthetic solution colored with methyl violet in a glass model that resembled the curves of the human spinal canal (Figure 3.6.5), and that gravity and the curvature were the main factors controlling the level of anesthesia. He subsequently adopted this principle of hyperbaricity to surgery of the perineal region (Figures 3.6.6). However, he did not label the method, and his pioneering work was largely ignored for several decades, particularly in German-speaking countries and France. Consequently, Japanese surgeons, being devoted to German surgery, were likely to be unaware of Barker's articles. Furthermore, Park referred to 124 articles written in English and German when writing his treatise,[8] but failed to mention Barker's papers. Thus, Professor Saito and Park are likely to have devised their technique independently of Barker, or to have reintroduced Barker's technique in a more accurate expression.

References and Remarks

1. Parmley RT. *Saddle Block Anesthesia*. Springfield, CC Thomas, 1955. p.4–5.
2. Roman–Vega DA and Adriani J. Prolonged Spinal Anesthesia. Description of a Simplified Technique for Nupercaine. *Surgery* 1945; 17: 524–32.
3. Lundy JS. *Clinical Anesthesia*. Philadelphia and London, WB Saunders, 1942. p.204.
4. Fink BR. History of Neural Block. In: Cousins MJ and Bridenbaugh PO. eds. *Neural Blockade*. (2nd. ed.) Philadelphia, J. B. Lippincott, 1988. p.11.
5. Jacob AK, Kopp SL, Bacon DR, and Smith HM. The History of Anesthesia. In: Barash PG, Cullen BF, Stoelting RK, and Cahalan M. eds. *Clinical Anesthesia*. (6th ed.) Philadelphia, Lippincott, Williams & Wilkins, 2009. p.20.
6. Park RS. Controlled spinal anesthesia by means of applied hyperbaricity. *J. Japan Surgical Society* 1940; 41: 678–82.
7. Park RS. Controlled spinal anesthesia using hyperbaric anesthetic solution. *J. Japan Surgical Society* 1941; 42: 805–64.
8. Reference 7. p.824–5.
9. Saito M. *Regional Anesthesia and General Anesthesia*. Tokyo, Gakujutsu Shoin, 1949. p.56–7.
10. Saito M. Spinal Nerve Blockade and Sacral *Anesthesia*. In: Ichikawa T, Fukuda T, and Kuji N. eds. *Surgical Operations and Anesthesia*. Tokyo, Kokuseido Shuppan, 1950. p.53–79.
11. Barker A. Clinical experiences with spinal analgesia in 100 cases and some reflections on the procedure. *British Medical Journal* 1907; 1: 665–74.
12. Barker A. A second report on clinical experiences with spinal analgesia. *British Medical Journal* 1908; 1: 244–9.
13. Barker A. A third report on clinical experiences with spinal analgesia. *British Medical Journal* 1908; 2: 45–5.

Chapter IV National and International Factors that Hampered Advances in Anesthesia before the End of the Pacific War

The phrase "before the End of the Pacific War" in the title of this chapter is an ambiguous expression. To be precise, it indicates the period between the latter years of the Taisho era (1912–1926) and the earlier years of the Showa era (1926–1989), i.e. the period approximately corresponding from 1919 to 1945.

During this period, remarkable advancements in anesthesiology were achieved in the United States and the United Kingdom, as evidenced by the introduction of endotracheal anesthesia (1920), CO_2 absorption system (1924), and closed circle system (1928) as well as the use of cyclopropane (1930) and thiopental (1934).[1,2] However, most Japanese surgeons ignored these advancements. Therefore, the practice of anesthesia in Japan became stagnant and outdated. Although the reasons why these American and British advancements in anesthesiology were ignored are briefly discussed in "The Blank 20 Years, 1925–1945" (slides 40–55) of chapter I and in chapter III, section 4 "The Blank 20 Years in the History of Anesthesia between 1925 and 1945 –The Lost 20 Years–," it will be difficult to correctly comprehend a perspective of the history of anesthesiology in Japan, if no information is provided to the reader regarding national political situations in Japan and several international difficulties, including the diplomatic tension between Japan and the United States during this period.

Among the 10 sessions on basic and clinical medical sciences presented at the Japanese–American Joint Conference on Medical Education in July 1950 in Tokyo, the session discussing advancements in anesthesia presented by Dr. Meyer Saklad, an anesthesiologist of Rhode Island Hospital, Providence, USA, substantially impacted the Japanese physicians in attendance. This fact clearly demonstrates that the academic and practical gap between Japan and the United States was actually greater in the field of anesthesiology than any other specialty and that modern American knowledge and anesthetic techniques were avidly desired by Japanese surgeons.[3–7] On this occasion, the Japanese neologism "*masui–gaku*" was coined to describe the specialty of "anesthesiology";[8] however, this term was inappropriate because it literally only refers to the "study of anesthesia." The term does not accurately convey the meaning of a clinical specialty. Therefore, the current author proposed that "*masui–gaku*" should be revised to "*masuika–gaku*" because the latter includes the meaning of both "science of anesthesia" and "clinical specialty" and is a more appropriate translation of "anesthesiology." This proposal was formally adopted by the Japanese Society of Anesthesiologists in 2001, and the Japanese title of the society was subsequently changed to "*Nihon Masuika Gakkai*."[9,10]

In 1951, the year after the joint conference, Wasaburo Maeda (1894–1979) (Slide31 of Chapter Ⅰ), a professor of surgery at Keio University, Tokyo, who had been the Japanese mediator of surgery and anesthesia sessions at the joint conference, delivered a presidential address entitled "We are in dire need of education and research in anesthesiology" at the 51st Annual Meeting of the Japan Surgical Society (JSS).[11]

In the final part of the introduction of his lecture, Maeda stated, "the descriptions of anesthesia in Japanese textbooks of general surgery are outdated and are behind the West by one generation. It is a serious problem that young surgeons lack the rudimentary knowledge of general anesthesia."[12] He continued to mention, "this severe situation has been caused by the dereliction of senior surgeons who are responsible for educating young surgeons and conducting research in the field of anesthesia." He concluded his lecture by stating following:

> The visit of Dr. Saklad last year was of remarkable significance to us because it sounded as an alarm to revive the practice of anesthesiology in Japan. First of all, we have to urgently introduce the American practice of anesthesia and then develop our own basic and clinical studies on anesthesiology. There are many research themes in anesthesiology to explore. I would like to urge our members to brace themselves.

His presidential address clearly indicated that Saklad's lecture had an enormous impact on the Japanese surgical community. Hideo Yamamura, an assistant surgeon at the First Department of Surgery of the University of Tokyo, was in the audience and enjoyed Saklad's lectures. Later, Yamamura became a professor of anesthesiology at the university and recollected Saklad's visit to Japan as that of Commander Matthew C. Perry's to Uraga Bay during the visit of the "Black Battle Ships" in 1853.[13] Saklad's impact was profound and significant to the Japanese surgical community and the overall field of Japanese medicine.

The considerable influence of Saklad's lecture on Japanese surgery can be exemplified by some specific figures. According to the current author's research,[14] approximately 100 Japanese physicians studied abroad during a relatively short 10–year period between 1951 and 1960 mainly in the United States to learn these advancements in anesthesia.[15] This period corresponds with the formative years in the history of anesthesia in Japan. Although the figure of 100 is not exact because it is difficult to document personal careers due to privacy issues, approximately 50 of these 100 physicians worked as qualified anesthesiologists in medical schools and major hospitals in Japan after completing their anesthesia training in the United States. Another 40 physicians not only from surgical departments but also from other departments, such as orthopedic surgery, and gynecology and obstetrics, returned to Japan and worked in their own departments as part–time anesthetists but were not qualified as anesthesiologists. The remaining 10 physicians remained in the United States as researchers or clinicians after completing their training.[16]

It is rather remarkable in the Japanese history of medicine that 100 physicians studied abroad only to gain knowledge and learn techniques in the relatively limited field of anesthesiology featuring tracheal anesthesia over a relatively short 10–year period. Almost the same number of surgeons studied abroad during the Meiji era (1868–1912) in 44 years.[17] In 1952, only two years after Saklad's visit, the first independent department of anesthesiology at the University of Tokyo, and in 1953, the foundation of the second department followed at Tohoku University, Sendai. In 1954, four years after Saklad's lectures, the former Japan Society of Anesthesiology was founded. Considering these advents, it is easy to understand the enormous impact that Saklad's lectures had on the modern Japanese medical community after the end of the war. Therefore, Saklad's visit was comparable with that of Commander Perry's "Black Battle Ships" for the post–Pacific War medical community in Japan.

This history clearly demonstrates that Japanese surgeons strongly desired further knowledge and techniques in general anesthesia featuring tracheal anesthesia in the 1950s. It also showed how their ardent desire for implementation of tracheal anesthesia was particularly strong among thoracic surgeons who were assiduously working on the surgical treatment of pulmonary tuberculosis, which was an epidemic among young persons at that time.[18] Reviewing this situation from a different perspective, the emergent need for modern techniques in general anesthesia was a reflection of the apparently outdated practice of anesthesia in Japan. It is necessary to elucidate the reasons for impeded advancements in anesthesia and to clarify the history of modern anesthesiology in Japan to gain an appropriate perspective on the specialty.

The issue of delayed progress in the practice of anesthesia in Japan before the end of the Pacific War should be discussed not only from the viewpoint of surgical specialty but also from that of the medical community as a whole. In addition, several topics should be considered from the various historical views of politics, diplomacy, social community, military affairs, liberal cultures, and medical politics. Because numerous pages would be required for detailed discussions of all of these considerations, only major factors are summarized in Table 4.1.1, and brief comments are made with minimum references.

Table 4.1.1   National and International Factors that Hampered Advances in Anesthesia in Japan before the End of the Pacific War

I   National Factors
  A The Japan Surgical Society
    1 Japanese Allegiance to German Surgery
    2 Concept of "Anesthesia" among Surgeons
    3 A Report from Miyake's Department at Kyushu University on Postoperative Mortality
    4 The Controversy on Thoracotomy
  B Japanese Medical Community
    1 The Japanese Association of Medical Sciences (JAMS)
    2 The Japan Medical Association (JMA)
  C The Ministry of Health and Welfare
  D The Ministry of Education
  E Pan–Asianism
II International Factors
  A World War I
  B Diplomatic Problems
    1 Naval Reduction Conferences
    2 Immigration Act of 1924
  C Sustained Standards of German Medicine after World War I

I **National Factors:** Continued allegiance to German medicine and unfavorable attitude toward American medicine

A The Japan Surgical Society (JSS)
1 Japanese Allegiance to German Surgery
Since the adoption of the German style of education, research, and patient care in medicine by the Meiji Government in 1870, almost all pioneering Japanese surgeons visited German–speaking countries to study surgery during the Meiji era (1868–1912), which were the formative years of the JSS. Since 1884, when Carl Koller from Vienna, Austria, first described the clinical use of the local anesthetic cocaine in ophthalmology, local and regional anesthesia rapidly developed in German–speaking countries. Consequently, it was only natural that Japanese surgeons who studied in these countries were much concerned with local anesthesia rather than general anesthesia. Thus, Japanese surgeons no longer studied general anesthesia and the anesthetic management of surgical patients,[19] although this practice continued throughout the country. This is exemplified by the fact that Kuhn's monograph on tracheal intubation[20] was not introduced in Japan despite the devotion of Japanese surgeons to German surgery, suggesting that Japanese surgeons preferred local anesthesia over general anesthesia.

Mishima[21] reviewed the history of surgery in Japan and concluded that Japanese surgery progressed to some extent after the period of exclusive devotion to the German system of surgery. However, advancements in Japanese medicine, including surgery, were severely impeded until after the end of the Pacific War because Japanese practitioners were isolated from their peers in the Western countries during World War II. A popular opinion among Japanese medical historians on the subject is that the delayed advancements in Japanese medical sciences emanated from the Pacific War. However, it is now clear that the delay in surgical advancements in Japan was not only caused by isolation from Western medicine or economic and material exhaustion due to the Pacific War but also by several much more important factors that are discussed later in this chapter.

Although the details about the surgery students who trained abroad during the period between 1919 and 1945 remain largely unknown, the general trend may be similar to that during the Meiji era, when most surgeons who studied abroad exclusively visited Germany and German–speaking countries.[22] For example, Seigo Minami (1893–1975), who later became a professor of dermatology at Kyushu University and was the first to describe "crush syndrome," traveled to Germany in 1922 and stayed there for two years.[23] In addition, Masao Muto, who later became a professor of surgery at Tohoku University and hosted the First Annual Meeting of the Japan Society of Anesthesiology studied in German-speaking countries from 1932 to 1934.[24] These two cases are mere examples to illustrate the trend of physicians and surgeons studying abroad during the Taisho and Showa eras, and most Japanese surgeons exclusively adhered to German surgery practices because they tended to consider American surgery second-rate and the practice of anesthesia only as a complement to surgery. They also considered the American practice of anesthesia as having the least significance. There were only three exceptional Japanese surgeons at the time who appropriately estimated American Anesthesiology: Hayao Nakatani of the First Department of Surgery at the University of Tokyo, Daisuke Nagae of the Army Medical School, and Kenji Tanaka of the First Department of Surgery at Niigata University.[25] The personal histories of these three surgeons are discussed in slides 45–55 in chapter Ⅰ and in chapter Ⅲ, section 5 "Hayao Nakatani, Another Surgeon who Appreciated Modern American Anesthesiology in the 1930s."

2 Concept of "Anesthesia" among Surgeons

In Japan, surgeons traditionally considered the performance of anesthesia as a relatively simple undertaking equal to "disinfection" techniques, and internists also deemed "anesthesia" a comparatively simple technique that was similar to "subcutaneous or intravenous injection."[26] These attitudes suggested that "anesthesia" was a relatively simple procedure to be performed by nurses but not by physicians. These viewpoints were widely accepted by lay people as well as physicians. Consequently, surgeons and internists shared the disdaining opinion that the practice of anesthesia could and should be performed by nurses. It was also a traditional concept that anesthesia itself was not directly connected with the diagnosis and treatment of certain diseases; rather, it was an ancillary measure for arriving at a diagnosis or for pain relief. In other words, the prevailing opinion at the time was that "anesthesia" was neither essential nor significant to the practice of medicine,[27] and there is no doubt that the opinion was widely shared by the general public in Japan. Under such circumstances, it was rational that no positive motivation emerged among young surgeons to further study "anesthesia" to improve anesthetic management or pain control for surgical patients during the intraoperative and postoperative periods. This situation is exemplified by the fact that there was no Japanese term for the "specialty of anesthesia" at that time.

Based only on the viewpoint that anesthesia was merely a technique of medical care and a complement to surgery, no physician, including surgeons, desired to specialize in the field. In Germany, whose system was used as the model of Japanese medicine since 1870, there were many surgeons who aggressively studied anesthetics and anesthetic methods, but none were specialized in the field prior to 1950. The same was true in Japan before 1950. Physicians began to specialize in anesthesia at the beginning of the 20th century in the United States and the United Kingdom, and societies were formed to exchange information and improve skills and social position. Shortly thereafter, independent departments were established at universities to train the next generation of anesthesiologists.[28] These advancements widely and profoundly promoted the study of basic and clinical anesthesia.[29, 30] In addition, it should not be overlooked that the modern practice of anesthesia rapidly began to advance in the United States beginning from ca. 1925,[31] coinciding with the time that surgeons began refraining from the use of general anesthesia in Japan.

3 A Report from Miyake's Department at Kyushu University on Postoperative Mortality

The topic is discussed in slides 41–43 in chapter I and in chapter III, section 4, "The Blank 20 Years in the History of Anesthesia between 1925–1945 – The Lost 20 Years –." This report demonstrated that postoperative mortality in patients with gastric cancer within one month of surgery decreased from 33.1% to 16.1% with the use of local anesthesia instead of general anesthesia. This was a shock to surgeons and a motivation to refrain from using and studying general anesthesia. It urged them to employ local anesthesia instead. This growing dissatisfaction with general anesthesia is clearly demonstrated by the number of presentations related to general anesthesia at the annual meeting of the JSS after publication of the report, as the proportion of presentations related to general anesthesia after publication decreased to 50% compared with the previous meeting.

4 The Controversy on Thoracotomy

This issue is also discussed in slide 41 of chapter I and chapter III, section 3. Together with the influence of the report from Miyake's Department, the debate over thoracotomy with or without positive–pressure ventilation which continued for more than 10 years beginning in 1925, apparently gave rise to a trend among surgeons to avoid general anesthesia with positive-pressure ventilation. There is no doubt that the motivation to study tracheal anesthesia was completely dissolved, although updated information was shared to Japan by Nakatani, Tanaka, and Nagae as early as the 1930s.

B Japanese Medical Community
1 The Japanese Association of Medical Sciences (JAMS)

The JAMS was founded in 1902; however, there is no definite proof demonstrating that this association actively accepted American medicine. The records of the annual meetings of the JAMS contain no description of American lecturers. At the 8th Meeting of the JAMS held in 1930, eight foreign guests presented lectures to the general assembly,[32] and among them, only one American biologist was included. Considering this fact, it is evident that there was no significant American influence on Japanese medicine as far as the JAMS was concerned. One possible explanation for the disregard for American medicine was the traditional opinion among Japanese physicians since 1870 that American medicine was second-rate to German medicine, and these viewpoints were likely reinforced by the fact that there were no American Nobel Prize laureates in the fields of Physiology and Medicine before 1930.[33]

The Third Pan-Pacific Science Congress was held in Tokyo in October 1926 and was partly hosted by several eminent members of the JAMS. The medicine-related presentations at the general assembly focused on the origins of human races in the Pacific areas and on specific diseases found in various races in the districts and their prevention and treatment. No lectures on American medicine were presented at the section meeting of medicine.[34]

2 The Japan Medical Association (JMA)

In 1916, the Great Japan Medical Association was founded as a national organization of practicing physicians. The first president of the association was Shibasaburo Kitasato (1853–1931), a bacteriologist and one of the discoverers of diphtheria and tetanus antitoxins. In 1919, according to the promulgation of the Medical Association Law, an association was to be found in each prefecture. Thereafter, the national Great Japan Medical Association was renamed the JMA, and Kitasato was again elected as the first president of this newly established association. In 1942, the Medical Association Law was revised because of the war, and in 1943, the JMA was dissolved and re-organized as the New Japan Medical Association. Under such rapidly changing circumstances, which were partly because of the war-time efforts, no trend arose among the executive members of the association or practicing physicians to improve the quality of patient care. Therefore, there was no basis to train physicians in the specialized practice of anesthesia.[35] In addition, there was neither an opportunity at that time for physicians to obtain information on modern American medicine nor a chance to introduce it into practice.

C The Ministry of Health and Welfare

There was no active movement in the Ministry of Health and Welfare to modify or improve the conventional system of medical education, research, and patient care that was based on the German system.[36,37] Although the issue of a qualification system for respective clinical specialties was stipulated in the National Medical Service Law (*Kokumin Iryo Ho*) adopted in 1942, according to the changes in designations of clinical specialties, further actions were postponed because of the war.[38]

D The Ministry of Education

The Ministry of Education showed an interest in the new American system of medical education, which began to emerge in the 1910s, as evidenced by the translation of 1910 report by A. Flexner[39] on medical education in North America and Canada.[40] Although this report recommended employing a style based mainly on clinical training, there was no implementation of such a program by the Ministry to improve the Japanese system of medical education.

In 1925, Emile Charles Achard (1860–1944), a French physician who discovered Salmonella paratyphi B, received an invitation to lecture in Japan from the La Maison Franco–Japonese and volunteers from the University of Tokyo. He presented lectures on the French system of medical education at several universities including the University of Tokyo. However, there was no discernable indication of his influence on medical education in Japan.[41] At that time, the Ministry of Education was confronted with a difficult problem with public medical schools being elevated to the status of a medical college. Therefore, at that time, it was not possible to make improvements to the conventional medical education system even by partially adopting the developing modern American or French educational system.[42]

E Pan–Asianism

In the field of liberal arts, there was a strong trend among the Asian countries from the 1920s to the 1930s for the independence of the Asiatic people.[43] Miyazaki,[44] a well-known historian of Kyoto University, described the following in his writing:

> "A national ambition of the Japanese people in the early years of the 20th century was to stand at par with the Europeans. Although the power of the Japanese military was partially recognized through the Qing–Japanese and the Russo–Japanese wars, Japanese economic and cultural standards were far behind those of the European countries. In hopes of overtaking the West in the field of literal arts, the Japanese became aware of the difficulty of this endeavor only through efforts of slavish imitation, which occurred during the "Cultural enlightenment" period in the early years of the Meiji Era. The Japanese became aware of the importance of improving the quality of their own culture to compete with Western cultures."

Miyazaki illustrated two examples, Unokichi Hattori's revision[45] of Koh Yasui's "*Rongo Shusetsu*" wherein Hattori used no honorifics to describe the behavior of Confucius and Jiro Izawa's annotation[46] of *the Analects of Confucius*, which was considered by Izawa as the gospel. In the deep intensions of Hattori and Izawa, it was likely that their real intentions were national awareness or Pan–Asianism. Their opinions were never interpreted as irresponsible remarks from anarchic intellectuals; rather, they solicited for the sympathy of the Asians and the confidence of the Japanese people.

A specific example of the effect of Pan–Asianism among the medical community can be detected in the *Encyclopedia of Medicine*, which was in publication since 1929.[47] Sawai[48] indicated that the publication was a standardizing movement for medical terminology in the early years of the Showa era, although the movement itself was likely to be a self–assertion of Japanese medicine in the context of Pan–Asianism. Ogawa,[49] a Professor Emeritus of Anatomy at the University of Tokyo, and a professor of medical history at Juntendo University thereafter, commented on this issue as follows:

> "The trend in the Japanese medical community of being dependent on Germany was gradually toned down during the course of World War Ⅰ, and Japanese medicine became independent during the Taisho era. It was not because Japan crossed swords with Germany in the Far East or that Germany and Austria met with a terrible defeat. It was because the Japanese people were awakened."

II International Factors

International factors impacting the delayed advancements in anesthesiology include tenacious devotion to German medicine and a disfavoring attitude toward the acceptance of American medicine.

A World War I

World War I broke out on July 28, 1914, when Austria and Hungary declared war on Serbia. Germany supported Austria as an ally, whereas Russia supported Serbia because of racial relatedness. Because Russia was allied with France, Germany proclaimed war against France, which eventually led to the participation of the United Kingdom in the war on the French side. In 1902, Japan concluded an alliance with the United Kingdom. Takaaki Kato (1860–1926), the Japanese Foreign Minister at the time, played a dominant role in the Japanese participation in the war because he was profoundly acquainted with British diplomacy through his experience as an envoy and ambassador to the Court of Great Britain. He finally decided to join the war in accordance with the Anglo–Japanese Alliance.[50,51] Thus, Japan entered the war against Germany on August 23, 1914. Qingdao, a territory in China leased by Germany, fell in November, 1914, after being shelled by the Japanese military, and the German islands north of the equator in the South Pacific Ocean were also occupied by the Japanese forces.

Because of Japanese participation in the war, the diplomatic relationships between Japan and Germany became nonexistent; thus, scientific exchanges were also interrupted. Japanese physicians who were studying in Germany and German–speaking countries were evacuated to other countries before returning to Japan. Because the war was worldwide and many of the involved countries became economically exhausted, there was no alternative for Japanese students to study abroad in other countries in place of Germany. Although the 5–year absence of cultural exchange due to the war from 1914 to 1919 had tremendously impeded advancements in German medical sciences, they were still considered to be of high standard throughout the world. In addition, the fact that more than 700 medical students had studied abroad mainly in Germany over a 44–year period between 1868 and 1912[52] indicated that the German system of medicine deeply permeated the Japanese medical community and that the leaders in the medical community could not afford to objectively observe scientific research in any other country other than Germany. In this sense, World War I caused an interruption on the academic exchange between Japan and Germany, although it was of short duration and its influence was minimal, at least when the subject is limited to the medical sciences.

   B Diplomatic Problems
   1 Naval Reduction Conferences

The Naval Reduction Conferences in Washington (1921–1922), Geneva (1927), and London (1930), were held during relatively peaceful years internationally, although political negotiations provoked a nationally heated confrontation between two factions in the Navy Ministry of Japan (i.e., a "pro-reduction group" and an "anti-reduction group"), which aggravated and intensified over the course of time. This internal situation was largely based on the ratio of the number of major warship, allowed according to an international agreement, i.e., 10 for the United States, 10 for the United Kingdom, and six for Japan or "60%" of the number permissible for the United States and the United Kingdom. This perceived imbalance provoked national emotions, accusing the United States and the United Kingdom of bestowing unreasonable demands on Japan, thereby generating a common repulsion among the Japanese against the United States.[53-55] In such an atmosphere, no emotion favoring the United States emerged among the Japanese people. Although it may be incorrect to assert that a trend to accept the evolving American practice of medicine did not develop among the members of the Japanese medical community, a result of the naval reduction talks tended to generate at least a negative effect on the emergence of such a trend. As mentioned in the "Japanese Medical Community," Japanese physicians continued to practice and support German medicine because of the anti-American sentiment of the citizenry.

   2 Immigration Act of 1924

One cannot deny that the Immigration Act instituted in 1924 in the United States had a grave impact on the relationship between Japan and the United States.[56-59] The act became widely known because Emperor Showa (1901–1989) suggested that it was the underlying cause of the Pacific War.[60] The Japanese public saw this law as an intentional and unbearable insult by the American Congress and was determined to protest against the act because it was considered an American prejudice against colored people. It is apparent that such national emotions had a significant impact on Japanese politics and diplomacy. It was also suggested that this likely effected to the boycotting of American medicine and its associated advancements by the Japanese medical community. In 1924, a report was presented from Miyake's Department at Kyushu University on postoperative mortality of patients with gastric cancer and a notorious debate began the next year among the members of the JSS on the subject of thoracotomy. In addition, it should be noted that remarkable advancements began in American anesthesiology in ca. 1925.[31]

C Sustained Standards of German Medicine after World War I

After the end of World War I, victorius nations and especially those that were defeated were severely exhausted in every aspect of social life. There was no question that this situation was most serious in Germany. Nevertheless, it should be noted that Germany maintained its high academic standards in the field of medicine, which can be illustrated by the number of Nobel Prize laureates in Physiology and Medicine after the war. The laureates by nationality during the period between 1919, when World War I ended and 1939 when World War II began, are as follows (in alphabetical order)[32]: three from Austria, two from Belgium, two from Canada, two from Denmark, one from France, four from Germany, one from Hungary, two from the Netherlands, five from the United Kingdom, and four from the United States. The fact that four laureates were from the United States, which had no laureate before 1930, clearly demonstrates the rapid evolution of American medicine over this period. Seven laureates were from German–speaking countries, which included four from Germany and three from Austria. Despite being defeated in the war, the medical standards in German–speaking countries remained first–rank in the world in terms of the number of Nobel Prize laureates in Physiology and Medicine, which inordinately fascinated Japanese physicians with the concept of superiority in the field.

References and Remarks

1. Keys TE. *The History of Surgical Anesthesia*. New York, Schuman's, 1945. p.114–6.
2. Rushman GB, Davies NJH, and Atkinson RS. *A Short History of Anaesthesia The First 150 Years*. Oxford, Butterworth–Heinemann, 1996. p.193–3.
3. Matsuki A. *A Short History of Anesthesia in Japan*. Hirosaki, Hirosaki University Press, 2012. p.161–6.
4. Maeda W. The Japanese American Joint Conference on Medical Education. –An impression of the surgery and anesthesia session–. *Geka* 1950; 12: 522–4.
5. Maeda W, and Takayama R. Anesthesiology in the United States–An impression of the anesthesia session at the Japanese–American Joint Conference on Medical Education–. *Shindan to Chiryo* 1950; 38: 664–8.

6. Shimizu K, and Yamamura H. Attending at the anesthesia session of the Japanese–American Joint Conference on Medical Education. *Rinsho Geka* 1950; 5: 481–6.
7. Kin–yokai. Attending at the Japanese – American Joint Conference on Medical Education. (A round–table discussion) –. *Sogo Igaku* 1950; 7: 1071–4.
8. It was in 1902 when Dr. M. J. Seifert from the University of Illinois coined the word *anesthesiology* and proposed Paul M. Wood, General Secretary of *American Society of Anesthetists*, to adopt this term because "an anesthetist is a technician and anesthesiologist is the scientific authority on anesthesia and anesthetics."
Collins VJ. *Principles of Anesthesiology*. (2nd ed.) Philadelphia, Lea & Febiger, 1976. p.25–6.
9. Matsuki A, Watanabe H, Kugimiya T, Odagiri T, Tsuda K, Hatano Y, Hirakawa M, and Terasaki H. eds. Chronology of Fifty Years of the Japanese Society of Anesthesiologists. *Masui* 2004; 53: S318–9.
10. Reference 3. p.15.
11. Maeda W. We are in dire need of education and research in anesthesiology. *J. Japan Surgical Society* 1952; 52: 566–8.
12. Refer to section 2 "Description of Anesthesia in Japanese Textbooks of General Surgery before 1949" in Chapter Ⅲ .
13. Yamamura H. Past and Perspective of Anesthesia in Our Country. *J. Jap. Soc. Clin. Anesthesia*. 1986; 6: 1–7.
14. Unpublished data.
15. The modern history of anesthesia in Japan begins with Saklad's visit to Japan in 1950. The 1st–5th presidents of the Japan Society of Anesthesiology (JSA, 1954–1958, the appellation was at the time) were professors of surgery, and Yamamura as a professor of anesthesiologist was the first president of the 6th Annual Meeting of the JSA in 1959. Therefore, 10 years from 1951 to 1960 are considered the formative years in the history of the specialty in Japan.
16. According to Hisayo O. Morishima, Emeritus Professor of Columbia University, 12 physicians and their affiliations are as follows.
    Kasumi Arakawa, Kansas University
    Luke M. Kitahata, Yale University
    Takako Kodama, practiced in San Francisco
    Kuwabara, practiced in San Francisco
    Hisayo O. Morishima, Columbia University
    Etsuro Motoyama, Pittsburgh University
    Hideo Nagashima, Monte Fiore Hospital
    Yasu Oka, Albert Einstein University
    Joe Shibutani, practiced in New York
    Kin–ichi Shibutani, New York Medical College
    Issaku Ueda, Utah University
    Name unknown, practiced in Hilo, Hawaii
17. Reference 3. p.117–30.
18. Miyamoto S. *My History of Surgery in the Showa era* (Watakushi no showa

geka–shi). Tokyo, Nihon Hyoronsha, 1985. p.76–88, 121–46.
19. Reference 3. p.130.
20. Kuhn F. *Die perorale Intubation*. Berlin, Karger, 1911.
21. Mishima Y. The Dawn of Surgery in Japan, with Special Reference to the German Society for Surgery. *Surgery Today* 2006; 36: 395–43.
22. Matsuki A. Studies abroad in the Meiji era and advances in anesthesia in Japan. In: Matsuki A. *The Acceptance of Anesthesiology and Its Development in Japan*. Tokyo, Shinkokoeki Ishoshuppanbu, 2011. p.117–43.
23. Matsuki A. Seigo Minami, the first to describe "Crush Syndrome" in the world. In: Matsuki A. *The Origin of Anesthesiology*. Tokyo, Shinkokoeki Ishoshuppanbu, 2006. p.208–19.
24. Muto M. A Glimpse of advances in anesthetic methods in the United States. *Tohoku Rinsho* 1951; 5: 76–9.
25. Refer to following references on three surgeons.
Hayao Nakatani: Section 5 "Hayao Nakatani, Another Surgeon who Appreciated Modern American Anesthesiology in 1930s" in Chapter Ⅲ
Daisuke Nagae: slides 45–50 in Chapter Ⅰ
Daisuke Nagae: Matsuki A. *A Short History of Anesthesia in Japan*. p.153–7.
Kenji Tanaka: slides 51–55 in Chapter Ⅰ
26. Amako S. ed. *Japanese Encyclopedia of Internal Medicine* (*Nihon Naika Zensho*). Tokyo, Tohodo, 1928.
    In the book, "anesthesia" was described as a technique equal to "antisepsis," "asepsis," "use of surgical instruments," "wound treatment," "injection," or "puncture." This clearly indicates that Japanese internists considered "anesthesia" as a technique in medical care.
27. A typical example is provided. When the division of anesthesia was formed in 1950 at the First Department of Surgery at the University of Tokyo, Dr. Akimi Uji–ie was asked to be a member of the division. He described the situation at that time as follows:
"I felt as if I were demoted from a commissioned officer to a noncommissioned officer."
Matuki A. *Unknown Episodes in the history of anesthesia in Japan* (*Postwar period*). Tokyo, Shinkokoeki Ishoshuppanbu, 2014. p.138.
28. They were called "anesthetist," and the term "anesthesiologist" was not yet coined at that time.
29. Reference 1. p.103–18.
30. Reference 2. p.201–2.
31. Larson MD. History of Anesthetic Practice. In: Miller RD. ed. *Miller's Anesthesia* (7th ed.). Philadelphia, Churchill Livingstone Elsevier, 2010. p.3.
32. According to the *Proceedings of the 8th General Meeting of the Japanese Medical Association* (Shotaro Takamura and Seiyo Yukawa eds. Osaka, the 8th General Meeting of the Japanese Medical Association, 1930), eight foreign guests and the titles of their lectures were as follows.
Thorvald Madsen (Copenhagen): Seasonal variation of infectious diseases
Theodor Axenfeld (University of Freiburg): Localization of intraocular

tuberculosis and juvenile angiopathy
Erich Hoffmann (University of Bonn): Is syphilis curable?
Charles Kofoid (University of California): Chronic amoebiasis
Etienne Burnet (Pasteur Institute in Tunis): Prevention of leprosy
Gaston Ramon (Pasteur Institute in Paris): Prophylaxis of diphtheria and immunization with anatoxine
Albert Calmette (Pasteur Institute in Paris): Preventive vaccination of tuberculosis with BCG
Nikolai Anitshkow (University of Leningrad): Pathogenesis of arteriosclerosis based on experimental and patho–anatomical study

33. www.nobelprize.org
34. Preparatory Committee. ed. *A Preliminary Report of Pan–pacific Academic Conference*. Tokyo, Preparatory Committee of the Pan–pacific Academic Conference, 1925.
35. Editorial Board of the Proceeding of the Committee on the 50 Years Anniversary of the Foundation of the Japan Medical Association. ed. *The 50 Year History of the Japan Medical Association after the Pacific War* (*Nihon ishikai soritsu kinenshi–sengo gojunen no ayumi*). Tokyo, Japan Medical Association, 1997. p.5–8.
36. Medical Affairs Bureau of the Ministry of Health and Welfare. (Koseisho Imukyoku) *Eighty Years History of Medical Care System in Japan* (*Isei hachijunen shi*). Tokyo, the Medical Affairs Bureau of the Ministry of Health and Welfare. 1955. p.171–8.
37. Medical Affairs Bureau of the Ministry of Health and Welfare. (Koseisho Imukyoku) *A Hundred Years History of Medical Care System in Japan*. (*Isei hyakunen shi*). Tokyo, Gyosei, 1976. p.190–2.
38. Kobayashi S. ed. *An Encyclopedia of Revised Medical Service Law and Related Regulations*. (*Kaisei iryoho kankei hoki zensho*). Tokyo, *Nihon Igaku Zasshi*, 1949. p.51–3.
39. The Ministry of Education. ed. *Medical Education in North America and Canada*. Tokyo, the Ministry of Education, 1918. p.51–3.
40. Flexner A. *Medical education in the United States and Canada: a report to the Carnegie Foundation for the advancement of teaching* (*Carnegie Foundation for the advancement of teaching No.4*). New York, Carnegie Foundation, 1910.
41. Kijima T. ed. *Collected lectures by EC Achard* (*Sharuru Asha–ru shi koenshu*). Tokyo, La Maison Franco–Japonese, 1926.
42. Amano I. The University Ordinance and medical student education in the Taisho and Showa eras. In Sakai T. ed. *A History of Medical Education in Japan* (*Nihon igaku kyoiku–shi*). Sendai, Tohoku University Press, 2012. p.149–85.
43. Yamamuro S. Crossing of Japanese diplomacy and Pan–Asianism (Nihon gaiko to ajia shugi no kosaku) In: Japanese Political Science Association ed. *Pan–Asianism in the Japanese diplomacy.* (*Nihongaiko ni okeru ajia shugi*). Tokyo, Iwanami, 1998. p.3–32.
44. Miyazaki I. *A new reading of the Analects of Confucius* (*Rongo no atarashii*

yomikata). Tokyo, Iwanami, 2000. p.267–71.
45. Hattori U. *Collected Annotations by Ko Yasui (Rongo Shusetsu* by Koh Yasui) (First volume of Kambun Taikei). Tokyo, Fuzambo, 1909.
46. Izawa J. *Rongo (The Analects of Confucius)*. Tokyo, Takemura Shobo, 1933.
47. *Modern Encyclopedia of Medicine* (27 volumes). Tokyo, Shunju Sha, 1929–33.
48. Sawai T. Medical terminology in medical education–its dissemination and standardization–. In: Sakai T. ed. *A History of Medical Education in Japan. (Nihon igaku kyoiku–shi)*. Sendai, Tohoku University Press, 2012. p.323–44.
49. Ogawa T. *A History of Medicine (Igaku no rekishi)*. Tokyo, Kodansha, 1964. p.214.
50. Inoue J. *World War I and Japan (Daiichiji sekai taisenn to nihon)*. Tokyo, Kodansha, 2014. p.12–59.
51. Hirama Y. *World War I and Japanese navy–Association of diplomacy and military affairs–(Daiichiji sekai taisen to nihon no kaigun–gaiko to gunji no rensetu–)*. Tokyo, Keio University Press, 1998. p.17–56.
52. Reference 3. p.117–8.
53. Kajima Institute of International Peace. ed. *The history of Japanese diplomacy16, the Naval Reduction Conference · Anti–war Treaty (Nihon gaikoshi 16 kaigun gunshuku kosho · fusen joyaku)*. Tokyo, Kajima Institute Press, 1973. p.6–77, 133–262, 263–361.
54. Mitani T. Democracy in the Taisho Era and Washington Regime 1915–30. In: Hosoya C. ed. *A regular history of Japan– United States relationship (Nichibei Kankei tsushi)*. Tokyo, University of Tokyo Press, 1995. p.77–109.
55. Asada S. *The Japan–American relationship during the two world wars–Navy and Processes of political decisions (Ryotaisenkan no nichibei kankei–kaigun to seisaku kettei katei)*. Tokyo, The University of Tokyo Press, 1993. p.149–204.
56. Kajima Institute of International Peace. ed. *The history of Japanese diplomacy13, the Washington Conference · Immigration Issue (Nihon gaiko shi 13 Washington kaigi · imin monndai)*. Tokyo, Kajima Institute Press, 1971. p.258–377.
57. Irie A. 1922–1931. In: May ER and Thompson JC. eds. *American–East Asian Relations: A Survey*. Cambridge, Harvard University Press, 1972. p.221–42.
58. Iminho Kenkyukai ed. *The World War II and Japanese immigrants (Senso to nihonjin– imin)*. Tokyo, Toyoshorin, 1997.
59. Minohara T. *The Immigaration Act in 1924 and Japan– American Relation (Hainichi iminho to nichibei kankei)* Tokyo, Iwanami, 2002.
60. Terasaki H and Miller MT. eds. *A monologue of the Emperor Showa–A daybook of Hidemasa Terasaki, a general affairs official of the Imperial Household– (Showa ten–no dokuhakuroku–terasaki hidemasa goyo gakari nikki)*. Tokyo, Bungei Shunju, 1991. p.20.

Chapter V History of Anesthesia in Japan after 1950

In this chapter, discussions focus mainly on four key events that triggered simultaneous advances in surgery and related specialties in Japan, symbolizing the beginning of the modern era of anesthesia in Japan after 1950. These events were (1) the lectures by Meyer Saklad at the Japanese–American Joint Conference on Medical Education (JAJCME) in Tokyo in 1950, (2) the establishment of the first independent department of anesthesiology at the University of Tokyo in 1952, (3) the foundation of the Japan Society of Anesthesiology (JSA) in 1954, and (4) the recognition of anesthesiology as a "specially approved designation" by the government in 1960. Understanding the origins of the practice of anesthesia and related specialties in Japan provides an important perspective regarding the history of the specialty

1   Meyer Saklad's Lectures at the JAJCME–according to Documents from Japanese and American Sources–

Among the lectures on basic and clinical medicines at the JAJCME, those by Meyer Saklad (1901–1979), an anesthesiologist from the Rhode Island Hospital, Providence, RI, U.S.A. had the most pronounced effect on Japanese professors. Because his influence on Japanese medicine was so great, his visit is often compared to that of Commander Perry to Uraga Bay in 1853.

The outlines and impressions of his lectures were assessed and

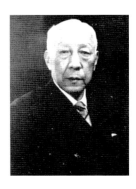

Figure 5.1.1   Wasaburo Maeda (1894–1979)

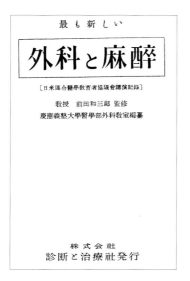

Figure 5.1.2 *The Newest Surgery and Anesthesia* published in 1951

subsequently introduced by some of the attendees immediately after the conference.[1-4] However, little was known about the detailed program of the lectures because, as of March 1987, no copy of the proceedings was available.[5] Moreover, I could not find them referenced in any medical libraries in Japan, including Kitasato Library of Keio University School of Medicine, where Professor Wasaburo Maeda (Figure 5.1.1), the editor of the proceedings, worked as the chairman of the Department of Surgery. In October 1987, after a nationwide survey for several years, I discovered a copy of the proceedings at the medical library of Kanazawa University. Here, the contents of this document are reproduced with permission from the Department of Surgery at Keio University.[6] They clarified that the proceedings entitled *The Newest Surgery and Anesthesia* (Figure 5.1.2) were published in January 1951, only 4 months after the JAJCME,[7] despite being thought to have only been published in 1952.

Recently, Ikeda[8] discussed Saklad's visit to Japan and described the contents of his lectures using the American documents of the visit. According to these documents,[9,10] the lectures in Tokyo began on July 25 and ended on August 8; however, the records for three days from July 19 to July 21 are omitted. The records included "General remarks for anesthetists," which was one of the most important parts of Saklad's lectures. The omission was probably because some members of the medical mission arrived in Japan several days behind the schedule. Therefore, the tentative opening ceremony was held on July 18 with only Professor Cyril N. H. Long and Dr. Meyer Saklad in attendance from the American team, and the formal opening ceremony only taking place on July 24. Consequently, the lectures delivered before July 23 were omitted from the formal American records, and only the lectures after that date were recorded, and later forwarded to the General Headquarters (GHQ) of the Supreme Commander for the Allied Powers. Here, I provide a reproduction of the exact daily schedule of the institute based on the records of the proceedings,[7] Maeda's report,[11] and the American documents[9,10]:

July 18 (Tue)	0900 :	Tentative opening ceremony, attended by Professor Long and Dr. Saklad
July 19 (Wed) Afternoon* :		① General remarks for anesthetists[12]
July 20 (Thu) Afternoon :		② Anoxia
		③ Oxygenation; its necessity during and after surgery, and its therapeutic effects
July 21 (Fri) Afternoon:		Instruments for oxygen therapy
July 25 (Tue) Morning** :		④ Education of anesthetists
		⑤ Premedication
		⑥ Pharmacology of anesthetic agents; general anesthesia
July 26 (Wed) Morning:		⑦ Inhalation anesthesia; practical methods of inhalation anesthesia. open–drop method, insufflation method, semi–closed method, to–and–fro method, closed–circle method, explanations of semi–closed method, to–and–fro method, and closed–circle method
July 27 (Thu) Afternoon:		⑧ Endotracheal anesthesia
July 28 (Fri) Morning :		⑨ Paradoxical respiration
July 31 (Mon) Morning:		⑩ Joint session with Professor Hoff; Origin and regulation of respiration
	Afternoon:	⑩ Joint session with Professor Hoff; Demonstration of new concepts of respiration in the dog
August 1 (Tue) Morning:		⑩ Joint session with Professor Hoff; Sensation with special reference to pain
August 3 (Thu) Morning:		⑩ Joint session with Professor Shafer; Anesthesia for thoracic surgery, and

156   Chapter V   History of Anesthesia in Japan after 1950

	anesthetic management of patients, pain relief, position during surgery, patient care during surgery, fluid replacement, oxygen supply, carbon oxide retention, influence on the vagus, and of the vago–vagal reflex
August 4 (Fri) Morning:	⑪Spinal anesthesia; theories on hypotension, nerve injuries, techniques in spinal anesthesia, toxicity and duration of action of local anesthetics, and patient care during spinal anesthesia
August 7 (Mon) Morning:	⑪Spinal anesthesia; segmental spinal anesthesia
August 8 (Tue) Morning:	Joint session with Professor Cattell; Analgesic agents
August 10 (Thu) Morning:	Closing ceremony

* : 1400–1700
** : 0900–1200

Number in circle:	corresponding to the same number of the contents in the proceedings.

Although I have described the simplified program of Saklad lectures, including the schedules for July 19 through July 21, they were not discussed in detail.[13] By using the reproduced daily schedules of Saklad's lectures, it is possible to provide a more exact review of this significant event.

It has also been stated that Saklad's lecture reached its culmination when he talked on endotracheal anesthesia in the afternoon of July 27. This was regarded as an exciting and stimulating day for the attendees, and it is also one of the more memorable days in the modern history of anesthesia in Japan. By collating documents from all involved countries, the details of such international advents are better illuminated.

References and Remarks

1. Maeda W and Takayama R. American anesthesiology–an impression of the anesthesia session at the Japanese–American Joint Conference on Medical Education. *Shindan to Chiryo* 1950; 38: 664–8.
2. Takayama R. American anesthesiology. *Igaku Tsushin* 1950; (222): 12–4

3. Shimizu K and Yamamura H. Attending at the anesthesia session of the Japanese–American Joint Conference on Medical Education. *Rinsho Geka* 1950; 5: 481–6.
4. Kin–yokai. Attending at the Japanese–American Joint Conference on Medical Education (a round–table discussion). *Sogo Igaku* 1950; 7: 1071–4.
5. As of 2015, only four copies of the first edition of the proceedings are extant in Japan as following: National Diet Library, Igaku Shoin Publishing Co., Medical Library at Kanazawa University, and the Japanese Museum of Anesthesiology.
6. Fujita T and Matsuki A. eds. *The History of Japanese Anesthesiology Source Material No3.*–Dr. Saklad and Japanese Anesthesiology–. Tokyo, Kokuseido Shuppan, 1989. p.47–170.
7. Maeda W. *The Most Recent Surgery and Anesthesia*. (1st ed.). Tokyo, Shindan to Chiryo Sha, 1951. The second edition was published in 1953.
8. Ikeda S. American Contributions to Japanese Anesthesiology–A Historical View –. *Masui* 2013; 62: 761–9.
9. Appendix A Schedule of Activities, Report of Institute on medical education Japan, July 19–September 5, submitted to General Douglas MacArthur by Dr. Cyril Long, Chairman, Unitarian Medical Mission to Japan 1950
10. Ikeda S. The Unitarian Serv ice Committee Medical Mission. Contribution by the United States to Post–World War II Japanese Anesthesiology. *Anesthesiology* 2007; 106: 178–85.
11. Maeda W. An impression of the surgery and anesthesia sessions at the Japanese–American Joint Conference on Medical Education. *Geka* 1950; 12: 522–4.
12. Because Japanese surgeons were unfamiliar with the term of "anesthesiologists," Professor Shimizu, the translator of the lecture, was likely to use "anesthetist (masui–i in Japanese)."
13. Matsuki A. *A Short History of Anesthesia in Japan*. Hirosaki, Hirosaki University Press, 2012. p.164.

2 Influence of Meyer Saklad's Lectures on Japanese Textbooks of Anesthesiology

Although Saklad's visit to Japan is often compared to Commander Perry's visit, and many articles have described Saklad's lectures at the JAJCME in 1950, no one has quantitatively evaluated the influence of his visit on Japanese anesthesiology.[1-5] In this section, the impact of his lectures on the evolution of anesthesia in Japan is, therefore, quantitatively assessed by means of languages and references cited in Japanese textbooks on anesthesia published before and after the lectures. It is conjectured that these textbooks reflect, to some extent at least, the trend in the practice of anesthesia at the time.

For purpose of this review, ten textbooks on anesthesia were selected (Table 5.2.1): five published before 1949 and five others published within three years of 1950. The latter were chosen because they were likely to reflect the direct influence of his lectures.

Three out of five textbooks published before 1949 are devoted solely to the topic of local anesthesia, demonstrating that local anesthesia was the predominant topic of anesthesia practice in Japan at that time. Although Miwa's textbook of 1916 includes two sections of anti–sepsis and asepsis, the descriptions of anesthesia cover 82.7% of total pages (291 of 352 pages), and provide more detailed descriptions than the other textbooks published before 1949. Takashima's textbook, published during the midst of the Pacific War in 1942, contains no references; however, foreign medical terms in the book were all in German. This is evidence of the practice of banning the use of English words by the Japanese medical community and the Japanese society during the war. This book is excluded from the statistical analysis because it contains no references, but evidences the influence of German practice on Japanese medicine. Among five textbooks published after 1950, *Surgical Operations* and *Anesthesia* edited by Ichikawa et al. was published in November 1950. Although much of these manuscripts were submitted to the publisher before Saklad's lectures, some of the authors provided their contributions after the lectures; thus it was suitable for inclusion as one of five "textbook after 1950."

In four textbooks published before 1949, excluding Takashima's book, no English–language references were found, while an average of 85.4% (range 66.7–100%) of all references was in German, and 14.6% were from Japanese source. These figures clearly demonstrate an apparent influence of German

Table 5.2.1 Languages of References cited in Japanese Textbooks of Anesthesiology published before and after Saklad's Lectures

Publication Year	Title	Author or Editor	Numbers and Languages of References (% in parenthesis)				
			English	German	French	Japanese	Total
1911	Local Anesthesia[1]	Miwa Y.	0(0)	142(100)	0(0)	0(0)	142
1912	Sacral and Lumbar Anesthesia[2]	Tongu	0(0)	10(66.7)	0(0)	5(33.3)	15
1916	General Therapy (General and Local Anesthesia)[3]	Miwa	0(0)	13(86.7)	0(0)	2(13.3)	15
1916	Local Anesthesia[4]	Kitamura K.	0(0)	67(88.2)	0(0)	9(11.8)	76
1942	Anesthetic Method[5]	Takashima R.	0(0)	0(0)	0(0)	0(0)	0
1950	Surgical Operations and Anesthesia[6]	Ichikawa T. et al eds.	15(53.6)	2(7.1)	0(0)	11(39.3)	28
1951	The Most Recent Anesthesiology[7]	Fukuda T. et al eds.	355(72.6)	51(10.4)	6(1.2)	77(15.7)	489
1952	New Anesthesiology[8]	Hoshiko N. Iwatsuki K.	10(31.3)	3(9.3)	0(0)	19(59.4)	32
1953	New Endotracheal Anesthesia[9]	Watanuki T.	28(71.8)	3(7.7)	1(2.6)	7(17.9)	39*
1953	Anesthesiology[10]	Amano M.	26(100)	0(0)	0(0)	0(0)	26

Remarks:
1. Miwa Y. *Local Anesthesia* (*Kyokusho masui*). Tokyo, Tohodo, 1911.
2. Tongu Y. *Sacral and Lumbar Anesthetic Method* (*Senkotsu oyobi yozui masuiho*). Tokyo, Nanzando, 1912.
3. Miwa Y. *General Therapy* (*General anesthesia, local anesthesia, antisepsis, and asepsis*) (*Ryoho soron, zenshin masui, kyokusho masui, seifuho, and bofuho*). Tokyo, Tohodo, 1916.
4. Kitamura K. *Local Anesthetic Method* (*Kyokusho mahiho*). Tokyo, Nankodo, 1916.
5. Takashima R. *Anesthetic Method* (*Masuiho*). Tokyo, Keibunsha, 1942.
6. Ichikawa T, Fukuda T, and Kuji N. eds. *Surgical Operations and Anesthesia* (*Shujutsu to masui*). Tokyo, Kokuseido, 1950.
7. Fukuda T, Araki C, and Shimizu K. eds. *The Most Recent Anesthesiology* (*Saishin masuigaku*). Tokyo, Igakushoin, 1951.
8. Hoshiko N, and Iwatsuki K. *New Introduction to Anesthesia* (*Atarashii masuigaku nyumon*). Tokyo, Kanehara, 1953.
9. Watanuki T. *Endotracheal Anesthesia and its precautions* (*Kikan-nai masui to sono chuiten*). Tokyo, Igakushoin, 1953.
10. Amano M. *Anesthesiology* (*Masuigaku*). Tokyo, Nankodo, 1953.

* A Latin reference is excluded.

medicine on the practice of anesthesia in Japan at the time. In the five textbooks published after 1950, the numbers of English references increased markedly reaching an average of 65.9% (range 31.3–100%) of all references. Meanwhile, German-language references decreased to an average of 6.9% (range 0–10.4%) and, by way of compensation for this decrease, Japanese literature increased to 26.5% after 1950.

There was, therefore, a remarkable increase in English-language references and the reciprocal decrease in German-language references in the anesthesia textbooks after Saklad's lectures. This exemplifies the fact that Saklad's lectures had a significant influence on the practice and education of anesthesia in Japan. Although the second Unitarian Service Committee medical mission visited Japan next year, and Professor Perry P. Volpitto gave lectures on anesthesia,[6] Yamamura commented that Volpitto had less marked effects than Saklad.[7]

References and Remarks

1. Yamamura H. Advances in Anesthesiology in Japan. In: Japanese Association of Medical Sciences. ed. *Proceedings of the 17th General Meeting of The Japanese Association of Medical Sciences*. Nagoya, Japanese Association of Medical Sciences, 1967. p.843–8.
2. Amano M. A History of Modern Anesthesia in Japan (1)–The 24–28 Years of the Showa –. *Rinsho Masui* 1977; 1: 10–9.
3. Yamamura H. Past and Perspective of Anesthesiology in Our Country. *J. Japanese Society for Clinical Anesthesia* 1986; 6: 1–7.
4. Fujita T and Matsuki A. eds. *The History of Japanese Anesthesiology Source Material No3.– Dr. Saklad and Japanese Anesthesiology –*. Tokyo, Kokuseido Shuppan, 1989. p.47–170.
5. Ikeda S. American Contributions to Japanese Anesthesiology–A Historical View–. *Masui* 2013; 62: 761–9.
6. Matsuki A. *A Short History of Anesthesia in Japan*. p.166–9.
7. Private communication with Professor Emeritus Hideo Yamamura. (May 16, 2014)

3   Professor Percival S. Bailey and Kentaro Shimizu –Seven Consecutive Chance Occurrences Leading to the Foundation of the First Department of Anesthesiology in Japan–

In the slide 55 of chapter Ⅰ of this book, the significance of Professor Percival S. Bailey's visit to Japan in 1948 was briefly discussed in association with the foundation of the independent Department of Anesthesiology at the University of Tokyo. In this section, further discussion is made to illustrate that there were seven consecutive chance events coincided in the foundation of the department at the university, beginning with Bailey's visit.

Kentaro Shimizu, who became the chairman and professor of the First Department of Surgery at the University of Tokyo, graduated from the university in 1929.[1] He joined the department chaired by Professor Tetsuzo Aoyama (1882–1953) in 1932 after receiving training in psychiatry and pathology. Shimizu was concerned with brain tumors and joined the department because Aoyama had reported two successful cases of the acoustic neurinoma removal.[2] In 1937, Shimizu reported an article in a German journal describing a refined method of cerebral angiography using percutaneous approach.[3] The method was appreciated by Professor Georges Schaltenbrand (1897–1979) of University of Würzburg, Würzburg, Germany, and his close friend Professor Percival Bailey of the University of Illinois also acknowledged Shimizu's paper and invited him as a research fellow in March 1940. Unfortunately, the Pacific War broke out in December 1941, and Shimizu together with the Japanese diplomatic officials and other Japanese people was forcibly taken in a hotel "Homestead" at Hot Spring, Virginia. From there they were repatriated aboard the Swedish passenger ship "Gripsholm" to Yokohama, Japan via Lourenço Marques (presently Maputo, Mozambique) in August 1942. Shimizu was promoted to an instructor at the First Department of Surgery at the University in January 1943 and then an associated professor in March 1945.

On August 24, 1948, Shimizu received a telephone call from the General Headquarters (GHQ), asking him to meet with Professor Bailey at the Imperial Hotel at 5 o'clock in the afternoon. It was quite an unexpected happening to Shimizu because he had not been informed of Bailey's visit beforehand. The exact reason for his visit to Japan remains unknown; however, it is certain that it was by the request of the GHQ, not the Japanese government, according to the records of Shimizu. This is the first of the chance occurrences.

Bailey's schedule was very tight because he had to do much work for the GHQ in a short time.[4] Shimizu met Professor Bailey for the first time in seven years, it must have been an excited meeting for both of them. Shimizu considered Bailey's visit an unequaled opportunity for a lecture, and asked him to give a lecture on neurology to Shimizu's Japanese colleagues. Bailey accepted his proposal, and after obtaining the GHQ's permission, delivered a lecture entitled "Recent Development in Neurology,"[5] which was held at the University of Tokyo on September 1. This is the second chance occurrence.

Despite being an unexpected and urgently held meeting, basic scientists, neurologists, and neurosurgeons who were interested in neurology attended from all over the country. At first, the lecture was to be given without interpretation; however, immediately before the lecture, Bailey asked Shimizu to translate it for better understanding. This was the third chance occurrence. The translation by Shimizu was an excellent opportunity for him to create an impression international recognition and English proficiency among the audiences, which included Professor Takeo Tamiya (1889–1963), the dean of the University of Tokyo Faculty of Medicine, and other professors of the university. With this opportunity supplying a tailwind, Shimizu was appointed professor and chairman of the First Department of Surgery in November 1948, only two months after the Bailey's lecture.

Professor Wasaburo Maeda from Keio University, who was later the Japanese mediator of the surgery and anesthesia sessions at the JAJCME in 1950, was also present at the lecture. This was the fourth chance occurrence because Maeda, who had known Shimizu's proficiency in English have asked Shimizu to translate Saklad's lecture at the anesthesia session two years later. The Slide 55 of Chapter I is a photograph taken just after Bailey's lecture in front of the auditorium of the University of Tokyo. Maeda is the first from the left in the front row and Shimizu, Kenji Tanaka, and Chisato Araki are placed second to fourth in the second row. These three were Professor Bailey's disciples.

During his visit, Bailey became aware that the study of neurology was outdated in Japan. After he returned to the United States, he asked the Rockefeller Foundation to supply the University of Tokyo with an electroencephalograph. The foundation decided to donate it to the Shimizu's department and asked him to send a technician to the United States to learn how to look after the instrument. Because no English–speaking candidate was eligible, and because Bailey had asked Shimizu to visit the Neurology Institute at the University of Illinois, Shimizu made his second visit to the United States in December 1949 and stayed there until July 1950. This is the fifth chance occurrence.

Shimizu was one of the Japanese physicians most familiar with modern American surgery because he had visited twice the United States before and after the Pacific War. Maeda, as the Japanese mediator of the surgery and anesthesia sessions may have corresponded with Shimizu to ask him to interpret Dr. Saklad's lectures at the anesthesia session because of Shimizu's proficiency in English. Shimizu returned to Japan on July 7, only 12 days before the start of the Saklad's lectures, for which Shimizu was the fluent interpreter. This is the sixth chance occurrence.

The need for an independent Department of Anesthesiology soon began to be recognized among Japanese professors of surgery. In response, Professor Muto of Tohoku University and Professor Shimizu both submitted applications to the Ministry of Education requesting the establishment of the Department of Anesthesiology. By coincidence, one of the high officers of the Ministry of Finance underwent a surgical operation at a private hospital run by Dr. Takeya Kikuchi, a member of the Shimizu's department. When the officer became aware of the importance of pain control during and after surgery, he suggested that an application for the Department of Anesthesiology would be financed if submitted. Kikuchi conveyed this message to Shimizu, who dutifully applied to the Ministry of Education to establish a Department of Anesthesiology.[6] This is the seventh chance occurrence. Thus, the first independent Department of Anesthesiology was founded at the University of Tokyo in 1952 based on a series of chance events.

References and Remarks

1. Matsuki A. Professor Kentaro Shimizu and the foundation of the Japan Society of Anesthesiology. In: Matsuki A. *The Roots of Anesthesiology*. Tokyo, Kokuseido Shuppan, 2005. p.63–75.
2. Aoyama T. Zwei operativ behandelte Fälle von Kleinhirnbrückenwinkeltumoren. *Deutsche Zeitschrift für Chirurgie* 1923; 178: 76–88.
3. Shimidzu K. Beiträge zur Arteriographie des Gehirns–einfache percutane Methode–. *Archiv für klinische Chirurgie* 1937; 188: 295–316.
4. Shimizu K. A diary of Dr. Bailey's visit to Japan. *No to Shinkei* 1948; (1): 69–70.
5. Bailey P. Recent Development in Neurology. *No to Shinkei* 1949; (1): 78–91.
6. Kikuchi T. An unknown episode of the foundation of the Department of Anesthesiology at the University of Tokyo. In: The First Department of Surgery of the University of Tokyo ed. *The Centenary Issue of the Foundation*

of the First Department of Surgery at the University of Tokyo (*The History of the First Department of Surgery, the fourth volume*). Tokyo, the First Department of Surgery of the University of Tokyo, 1993. p.274.

4   When Did Kentaro Shimizu Determine to Establish the Department of Anesthesiology?

In every field of natural and liberal science, even a small organization is essential for establishing the basis for the field and for promoting its development. In other words, meaningful progress is not possible without a dedicated organization; in a university, an independent department provides such a basis. Therefore, the foundation of the first independent Department of Anesthesiology at the University of Tokyo in 1952 was one of the most significant events in the history of anesthesia in Japan and was important to the advent of modern medical science in Japan.

In the previous section, the background to the foundation of the first independent Department of Anesthesiology at the University of Tokyo was described. It is apparent that the lectures by Meyer Saklad at the JAJCME in 1950 were critical. Professor Shimizu was the translator for Saklad at the anesthesia session of the JAJCME, and Shimizu was asked by Wasaburo Maeda of Keio University to do so before Shimizu came back to Japan on July 7, 1950 from his second visit to the United States.

Shimizu was most concerned with neurosurgery and was enthusiastic to establish an independent Department of Neurosurgery at his university. In fact, in January 1951, he established an outpatient clinic of neurosurgery at the university hospital. This was the first such clinic in Japan, and it developed later to the first independent Department of Neurosurgery in Japan in December 1962.[1]

On establishing the Department of Anesthesiology, Shimizu nominated Hideo Yamamura, an assistant at the First Department of Surgery as a candidate to chair the department because Yamamura had been the chief of the "anesthesia group" in the department since September 1950. In 1952, because he was too young (32 years old) to be a chairman and professor, Yamamura was promoted to associate professor and appointed the acting chairman of the newly founded Department of Anesthesiology. Thus, the origin of the first independent Department of Anesthesiology in Japan dates back to the "anesthesia group" at the First Department of Surgery of the University of Tokyo. According to Yamamura, the group consisted of four members, including Yamamura, and three others recruited from young members of the department every few months.[2] Thus, it can be said that the group was intradepartmental, but not interdepartmental. Every surgical department in Japan had their own independent operation theaters and informal anesthesia groups at this time. Shimizu's recognition of the need for the anesthesia groups to reflect American system of organization into departments of anesthesia is, therefore, significant to the history of anesthesia in Japan.

In a correspondence with myself, Yamamura[2] wrote that Shimizu was first cognizant of the importance of anesthesiology during his interpretation of Saklad's lectures in July 1950 because Saklad repeatedly emphasized the importance of the specialty. Indeed, Shimizu appreciated the rapid advancement in anesthesia in the United States during his second visit to the country between December 1949 and July 1950; it is understood that he gained a deeper and broader comprehension of American anesthesiology practice than any other Japanese surgeons and physicians of the time. This is substantiated by his comments at the editors meeting of the journal *Geka* held on July 18, 1950, only a day before the first lecture by Saklad,[3] where Shimizu[4] states:

> Lastly, advancements in surgery in Japan will be retarded without simultaneous progress in anesthesia. Developments in surgery are dependent solely on the evolution in anesthesia.

Shimizu had appropriately realized the importance of anesthesia before the joint conference, and his opinion of this subject was likely fortified by the lectures. This is exemplified by his comment on the subject. In an article on the anesthesia session that appeared in a journal in October 1950, Shimizu[5] wrote:

> Dr. Saklad kindly promised to support us as much as possible, if we are going to establish a new independent department of anesthesia. It may be impossible to set up the new department soon; however, we are planning to take a step of some sort before founding the department.

The "step of some sort" that Shimizu referred to was the formation of the "anesthesia group." Shimizu and Yamamura[6] also read a paper announcing the start of the anesthesia group at the 492nd Tokyo Surgical Society Conference held on November 17, 1950. In the presentation, Yamamura asserted that he had converted from a surgeon to an anesthesiologist. This announcement had an unexpected and considerable impact on every surgeon in attendance. Two surgical departments existed in every university and medical college across Japan, each with their own operating theaters;

therefore, there was a *de facto* "anesthesia group" in each department. However, the group usually comprised several novice surgeons, not of anesthesiologists, and they had no adequate mentors. Yamamura's resolution was therefore greeted with surprise and became the topic of debate among surgeons.[7]

It was in the middle of March 1950 when the Unitarian Service Committee decided to send a medical mission to Japan. This was in response to the request of the GHQ which accepted an urgent proposal of Yoshio Kusama (1888–1968), a professor of public health at Keio University and the chairman of the Council of Medical Education of the Ministry of Education. Kusama visited the United States from October 1949 to February 1950 to study American medical education system, and was aware of the success of the Unitarian Service Committee in Europe.[8] Immediately after returning to Japan, he met Crawford F. Sams (1902–1994), a brigadier general of the GHQ, asking for the Unitarian Service Committee to send a medical mission to Japan.[9] Sams and Kusama were alumni of the Stanford University School of Medicine. Consequently, the mission's visit was immediately settled in March 1950, and the members were decided by the end of the month.[10] Kusama and Maeda (the mediator of the surgery and anesthesia sessions), were working for the same university, which allowed rapid communication of the information that the mission would be composed of ten members and Saklad from the Rhode Island Hospital would be one of the members, giving lectures on anesthesiology. Maeda may have communicated with Shimizu in the United States, asking him to interpret for Saklad because no other surgeon was available with equivalent English–language proficiency in the new genre of anesthesiology. Shimizu's fascination with neurosurgery also meant that he was aware of the indispensability of both general and local anesthesia, for the management of patients undergoing neurosurgical procedures. This idea had been proposed by Professor Frazier of the University of Pennsylvania since the beginning of the 20th century,[11] and this was a traditional and prevailed opinion in American neurosurgery.

Considering these circumstances, Shimizu probably had the beginnings of the idea to establish Departments of Neurosurgery and Anesthesiology by the former month of 1950 during his second visit to the United States.

References and Remarks

1. Sano K. Kentaro Shimizu. *Brain Medical* 1994; 6: 101–3.
2. Private communication with Professor Emeritus Hideo Yamamura. (January

9, 2014)
3. Refer section 1 of this chapter. Because some members of the mission arrived behind the schedule at Japan due to the outbreak of the Korean War, the formal opening ceremony was postponed to July 24, but the first lecture by Saklad was given on July 19.
4. Shimizu K, Fukuda T, Ichikawa T, and Kuji N. A round–table discussion with Professor Shimizu as the main guest (1). *Shujutsu* 1950; 6: 488–91.
5. Shimizu K and Yamamura H. Attending the Japanese – American Joint Conference on Medical Education. *Rinsho Geka* 1950; 5: 481–6.
6. Shimizu K and Yamamura H. Some experiences with anesthesia. An abstract of the 492nd Tokyo Surgical Society. *J. Japan Surgical Society* 1950; 53: 113–4.
7. Kin–yokai. Attending at the Japanese–American Joint Conference on Medical Education (a round–table discussion). *Sogo Igaku* 1950; 7: 1071–4.
8. Anonym. Articles. Newspaper of Keio University School of Medicine (*Keiogijukudaigaku igakubu Shimbun*) October 10, 1949 and January 10, 1950.
9. Matsuki A. *A Short History of Anesthesia in Japan*. p.162.
10. Matsuki A. *Unknown Episodes in the history of anesthesia in Japan* (*Postwar period*). Tokyo, Shinkokoeki Ishoshuppanbu, 2014. p.142–4.
11. Frazier CH. Problems and procedures in cranial surgery. *JAMA* 1909; 52: 1805–13.

5 Establishment of the First Department of Anesthesiology and Foundation of the Japan Society of Anesthesiology

Table 5.5.1[1] illustrates the foundation years of various societies of anesthesia and the establishment of the first chairs of anesthesia in several foreign countries as well as in Japan. It is apparent that the societies of anesthesia in the foreign countries had been founded before the first chairs had been established. In contrast, the first independent Department of Anesthesia had been established at the University of Tokyo in 1952, before the Japan Society of Anesthesiology (the former appellation) (JSA) was founded in 1954. Thus, the first anesthesiology department preceded the foundation of the JSA, and contrasting with the typical pattern in other countries.

So, why did this dissimilar phenomenon occur in Japan? In Western countries, some physicians devoted themselves to the practice of anesthesia from the end of 19th century because they considered that the administration of general anesthetics required wide pharmacologic knowledge of the agents and skillful expertise in administering them. Moreover, they argued that the practice was neither a compliment to surgery nor a side job of a surgeon. Then, they gathered to discuss and exchange their knowledge and refine their skills, and formed societies for mutual communication and to raise

Table 5.5.1 Years of Foundation of Societies and Establishment of Chairs

	Societies			Chairs		
Country	Year	Designation	Year	University	Professor	
United Kingdom	1893	London Society of Anaesthetists	1937	Oxford	Robert R. Macintosh	
United States	1905	Long Island Society of Anesthetists	1933	Wisconsin	Ralph M. Waters	
Australia	1934	Australian Society of Anaesthetists	1962	Sydney	Douglas Joseph	
Italy	1934	Italian Society of Anesthesia and Analgesia	1962	Turin	Enrico Ciocatto	
Canada	1943	Canadian Anaesthetists' Society	1945	McGill	Wesley Bourne	
South Africa	1943	South African Society of Anaesthesiologists	1959	Pretoria	Ordino V.C. Kok	
Germany	1953	Deutsche Gesellschaft für Anaesthesiologie und Wiederbelebung	1960	Mainz	Rudolf Frei	
Japan	1954	Japan Society of Anesthesiology	1952	Tokyo	Hideo Yamamura[*]	

[*]: Yamamura was appointed as the chairman and associate professor.

their social position. Specialist anesthesiology departments then emerged in these countries, to educate physicians, and increase future membership at universities, with young members actively recruited. In contrast, in Japan, most surgeons considered the practice of anesthesia a supplement to surgery before Saklad gave his lectures at anesthesia session in 1950. Indeed, anesthesiology was considered a simple technique that could be done by a novice surgeon, or a trivial caring measure to be provided by a nurse. Consequently, there was no appetite to form a society in Japan.

This distressed situation was improved by Saklad's lectures in 1950, when Japanese professors of surgery comprehended the significance of anesthesia for advancement of surgery and began to ask young surgeons to work on basic and clinical studies of anesthesia.[2] Subsequently, the number of anesthesia-related papers at the annual meetings of the Japan Surgical Society (JSS) increased markedly (Table 5.5.2). A similar, but more pronounced trend was also observed in the numbers of anesthesia-related presentations at the annual meetings of the Japanese Association for Thoracic Surgery (JATS). Some executive members of the JATS were

Table 5.5.2 Numbers of Free Papers and Anesthesia-related Papers at the Annual Meetings of the Japan Surgical Society and the Japanese Association for Thoracic Surgery before and after Saklad's Lectures*

	Year No of Papers	1947	1948	1949	1950	1951	1952	1953	1954
JSS	Free Paper (A)	31	65	60	56	113	61	84	133
	A-related Paper (B)**	0	2	0	2	7	6	2	12
	B/A (%)	(0)	(3.1)	(0)	(3.6)	(6.2)	(9.8)	(2.4)	(9.0)
JATS#	Free Paper (A)	No	23	76	44	111	142	170	183
	A-related Paper (B)**	Meeting	0	0	0	8	13	16	0
	B/A (%)		(0)	(0)	(0)	(7.2)	(9.2)	(9.4)	(0)
JSA	Free Paper (A)								82
	A.-related Paper (B)*								82
	B/A(%)								(100)

*: modified from Table5.4.1 and Table 5.4.2. of *A Short History of Anesthesia in Japan* (2013)
**: Anesthesia-related paper
#: The first annual meeting of the Japanese Association for Thoracic surgery was held in 1948.
    JSS : the Japan Surgical Society
    JATS : the Japanese Association for Thoracic Surgery
    JSA : the Japan Society of Anesthesiology

anxious that if more anesthesia–related papers were submitted for the annual meetings of the JATS, the schedule would be too tight. To avert this, they concluded that a separate society should exist in which anesthesia–related papers could be exclusively read. Thus, the JSA was founded in 1954 by thoracic surgeons rather than by anesthesiologists, not least because only two anesthesiologists existed in Japan at that time (Hideo Yamamura, an associate professor of the University of Tokyo and Michinosuke Amano, an instructor of Keio University).[3] This is the most pronounced difference between Japan and other countries as far as the foundation of anesthesiology societies is concerned. Without understanding this background, it is difficult to appreciate the early history of modern anesthesia in Japan.

References and Remarks

1. Modified from Table 5.4.1 and Table 5.4.2 in Matsuki A. *A Short History of Anesthesia in Japan*. p.174–5.
2. Matsuki A. *The Origin of Anesthesiology, continued*. Tokyo, Shinkokoeki Ishoshuppanbu, 2009. p.79–101.
3. Matsuki A. *A Short History of Anesthesia in Japan*. 2013. p.173–4.

6   The First Tracheal Anesthesia for Surgery in Japan

The introduction of tracheal anesthesia has formed a major landmark in the history of anesthesiology in Japan. The process of tracheal anesthesia was formally conveyed to Japan in 1950 by Meyer Saklad at the JAJCME;[1] however, little was known about the fact that several ambitious surgeons of the University of Tokyo had devised a simple anesthesia machine immediately before Saklad's lectures and had developed independently the technique of tracheal anesthesia for surgery. Although several authors have described that the first tracheal anesthesia was administered in 1950, the exact date of the event is varied and confusing.[2-5] I, therefore, investigated this topic carefully because "the first" is of great concern in the study of history; however, this episode remains unknown, particularly to historians of Western medicine.[6,7]

As of 1950, Shuichi Hayashi (1916–2009) (Figure 5.6.1) and Tetsu Watanuki (1918–1980) (Figure 5.6.2) were members of the Second Department of Surgery at the University of Tokyo, chaired by Professor

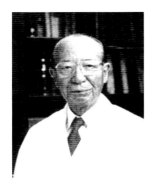

Figure 5.6.1   Shuichi Hayashi (1916–2009). With kind permission from Shuichi Hayashi.

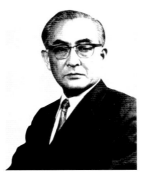

Figure 5.6.2   Tetsu Watanuki (1918–1980). Taken from *Memorial issue of the list of Professor Tetsu Watanuki's achievements*, published in 1983.

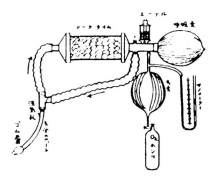

Figure 5.6.3 The prototype anesthesia machine by Hayashi. Taken from Reference 7.

Tamotsu Fukuda (1892–1974). Hayashi graduated from the University of Tokyo in 1941 and joined the same department presided over by Professor Masao Tsuzuki (1892–1961). Tsuzuki resigned the position in 1946 because he had been a naval rear admiral during the Pacific War, was succeeded by Fukuda. During the war, Hayashi worked for the Kure Naval Hospital, Kure, Japan, and returned to the department. Watanuki graduated from the same university in 1942 and joined the same department. He worked at field hospitals during the war and returned after the war was over. Both surgeons began studying tracheal anesthesia because they had to treat pulmonary tuberculosis surgically, which was prevalent among young men at that time. Local anesthesia supplemented with incremental doses of morphine was the standard practice for lung surgery, but was often unbearably tortuous for patients. Because they knew the effectiveness of tracheal anesthesia in pulmonary surgery, they began studying tracheal anesthesia in the beginning of 1949. They had a basic understanding of tracheal anesthesia by referring to a monograph by Adriani,[8] and started to manufacture a primitive anesthetic machine (Figure 5.6.3), and prepared a coiled metallic tube to substitute for a rubber tracheal tube, and crude soda lime. They began successful animal experiments in April 1950, and later, they refined the machine several times (Figures 5.6.4–6). Before clinical application of tracheal anesthesia, they had to master the technique of tracheal intubation from Jo Ono (1898–1988), a visiting professor of otorhinolaryngology at Keio University who was a graduate of Jefferson Medical College in 1928 and one of the leading disciples of Chevalier Jackson (1865–1958). Ono was also one of the most eminent pioneers in laryngoscopy in Japan. Watanuki mastered the technique of intubating the trachea from him.

According to Hayashi, tracheal anesthesia was first administered in May

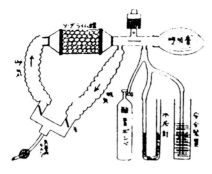

Figure 5.6.4 Revised anesthesia machine(2). Taken from Reference 7.

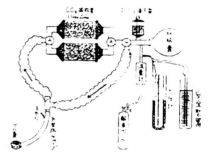

Figure 5.6.5 Revised anesthesia machine(3). Taken from Reference 7.

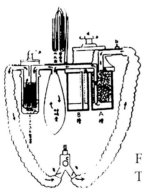

Figure 5.6.6 Revised anesthesia machine(4). Taken from Reference 7.

1950,[9] while his colleague Watanuki described that it was in June 1950.[10] Although there is a discrepancy of a month, Hayashi clearly remembered that they administered tracheal anesthesia for two surgical patients: a breast cancer patient in the morning and a gastric patient in the afternoon. To specify the exact date of the first tracheal anesthesia in Japan, I asked for

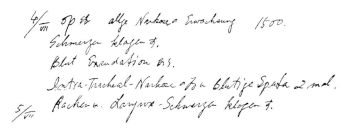

Figure 5.6.7　Admission record of Yasu Kawanishi (July4,1950).

cooperation of Dr. Hayashi and the Second Department of Surgery at the University of Tokyo. They kindly permitted me to investigate the relevant admission and discharge records, the operation registers, and patients' histories.

In the operation registers of May and June, 1950, there was no description of breast cancer and gastric cancer patients being treated on the same day, substantiating the fact that the first tracheal anesthesia was unlikely to have been performed in those months. Therefore, the descriptions by Hayashi[9] and Watanuki[10] were both incorrect. In addition, there is no possibility that the first tracheal anesthesia was administered in April because they only started animal experiments with tracheal anesthesia in this month, and because no operations were performed for breast and gastric cancer in one day during April. However, reviewing the records of July 4, 1950, both breast and gastric surgeries were performed under general anesthesia, and the records clearly described that the patients received tracheal anesthesia, with no other comparable days.

Yasu Kawanishi, a 50-year-old female from Tokyo, was referred by Hiroshi Kumagai and Tsuyoshi Sato (later Tsuyoshi Toyo-oka), and admitted on July 2, 1950 for amputation of the left breast, ipsilateral lymphadenectomy, and biopsy of the right breast. She received premedication with a 1 mL subcutaneous injection of Pantopon (opium derivatives) at 0930 hours on July 4 and the procedure was performed by Associated Professor Seiji Kimoto, taking 35 minutes from 1020 to 1055 hours. Her admission record for that day is shown in Figure 5.6.7. They are written in German phrases with Japanese prepositions, and their English translation reads as follows:

July 4th.　After general anesthesia [she was] awaken at 1500.
　　　　　Complained of [incisional] pain.
　　　　　Bloody exudation [observed] .

Bloody sputa expectorated 2 times because of intra-tracheal narcosis
Complained of pharyngeal and laryngeal pain.

The phrase "intra-tracheal narcosis" provides further evidence that this patient received tracheal anesthesia. There is no description as to who intubated the trachea of the patient, but Watanuki was the most likely candidate because he was most adept in the department. Despite the short duration of the surgical procedure, the patient took approximately four hours to awaken because the use of ether (at that time ether was the only inhaled anesthetic available). It was likely that, because this was the first clinical case of tracheal anesthesia and no muscle relaxants were available, Hayashi and Watanuki gave the patient a deep ether anesthesia to allow them to intubate the trachea. This may explain the patient's protracted recovery from anesthesia. Furthermore, the patient complained of postoperative pharyngeal and laryngeal pain, suggesting that either the metallic tube or Watanuki's immature intubation skills were responsible. Her admission record of July 5 (Figure 5.6.8) reads as follows:

> July 5th. Last night's sleep [of the patient] was disturbed due to incisional pain. Professor's round [was made]. Much bloody exudation [was observed], a bandage dressing changed. A rubber drain taken out [from the incision site], and a rubber tube taken from the right breast. [The patient] spit out bloody sputa two times due to tracheal anesthesia, and she complained of the sore pharynx and larynx with hoarseness. [The patient] was suffering from incisional pain all day.

This record describes the complications experienced on the first postoperative day, which apparently indicated they were originated from

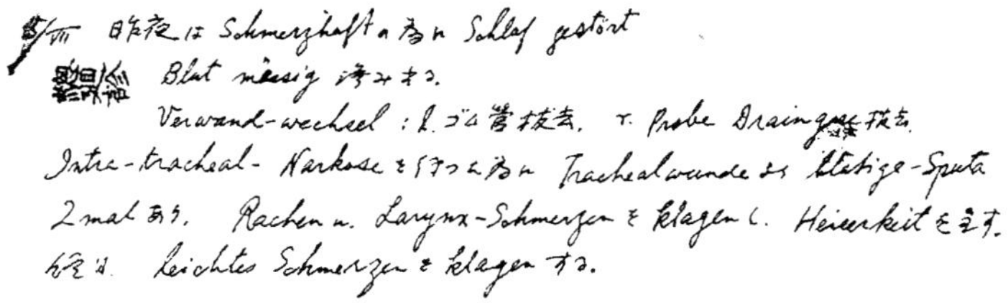

Figure 5.6.8　Admission record of Yasu Kawanishi (July5,1950).

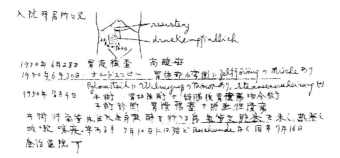

Figure 5.6.9 Admission record of Zensuke Ichiyanagi (July17).

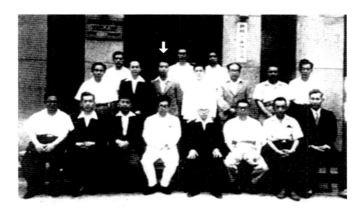

Figure 5.6.10 A photograph taken in front of the Research Institute for Tuberculosis and Leprocy of Tohoku University on July 20, 1950. With kind permission from Shuichi Hayashi. An arrow mark indicates Shuichi Hayashi.

tracheal intubation. She discharged uneventfully on July 17.

Zensuke Ichiyanagi, a 50-year-old man with gastric cancer, from Kamakura, Kanagawa Prefecture, underwent a gastrectomy in the afternoon of the same day (from 1350 to 1640 hours). His referring surgeons were Eikichi Orimo and Chiaki Iwase, and the operating surgeon was Orimo. A gastrectomy with gastro-jejunostomy was performed as illustrated in Figure 5.6.9. The third line from the bottom in the figure demonstrates that the patient developed postoperative broncho-pneumonia because of "intra-tracheal Narkose." Iwase was likely to use this bizzare phrase because the technique of tracheal anesthesia was unfamiliar to him. Nevertheless, the patient was discharged uneventfully on July 16.

Hayashi read a paper on these two cases on July 20 in Sendai, Japan, at a meeting of Surgical Treatment of Pulmonary Tuberculosis sponsored by the Ministry of Education (Figure 5.6.10). This was on the third day of the lectures by Saklad in Tokyo.

According to my investigation, it is therefore clear that Hayashi and Watanuki of the Second Department of Surgery of the University of Tokyo, performed the first tracheal anesthesia in Japan on July 4, 1950.

I acknowledge the late Shuichi Hayashi and Dr. Hitoshi Matsunaga (the director of the Hayashi Surgical Hospital, Tokyo) for providing invaluable information and photographs in support of this finding.

References and Remarks

1. Refer section 1 of this chapter.
2. Ishikawa S. Advances in thoracic surgery–anesthesia–. *Kyobu Geka* 1957; 10: 697–701.
3. Miyamoto S. The history of anesthesia in thoracic surgery–anesthesia for thoracic surgeons (1). *Kyobu Geka* 1972; 25: 26–8.
4. Amano M. A history of modern anesthesia in Japan (1) –the 24–28th Years of Showa–. *Rinsho Masui* 1977; 1: 10–9.
5. Yamamura H. History of anesthesia. In: Inamoto A, Iwatsuki K, and Yamamura H. eds. *Encyclopedia of anesthesiology*. Vol. I–1. Tokyo, Kanehara, 1969. p.7.
6. Matsuki A. Recent information on the first endotracheal anesthesia in Japan –achievement by Hayashi S. and Watanuki T.–. In: Fujita T and Matsuki A. eds. *The Japanese History of Anesthesiology. Source Materials No3*. Tokyo, Kokuseido Shuppan, 1989. p.140–52.
7. Matsuki A. A view on the first endotracheal anesthesia in Japan–achievement by Hayashi S. and Watanuki T.(revised). In: *Matsuki A. Unknown Episodes in the history of anesthesia in Japan* (*Postwar period*). Tokyo, Shinkokoeki Ishoshuppanbu, 2014. p.107–26.
8. Adriani J. *Techniques and Procedures of Anesthesia*. Springfield, Charles C Thomas, 1947.
9. Hayashi S. Memoirs of those days when we were beginning the research on tracheal anesthesia. *Masui* 1956; 5: 592–4.
10. Watanuki T. *Endotracheal anesthesia and its precautions*. Tokyo, Igakushoin, 1953. preface. p.1.

7 The Origin of "Specially Approved Designation" of Anesthesia and Board Certified Anesthesiologists

The origin and evolution of any scientific field inevitably depend on three elements: the numbers of researchers who devote themselves into the study of their field, the formation of a group or a society to exchange opinions and refine techniques, and a system of social support. Specifically, these involve the establishment of a university (college) or an institutional department, the foundation of a society or meeting, and the creation of a social guarantee system, respectively. As far as medical care is concerned, the third element, or provision of a public medical care system, is indispensable because it is so closely associated with people's health care and welfare.

One of the most remarkable events in the history of medicine after the end of the Pacific War in Japan was that the JSA launched the first qualification system in 1962 preceding those of other medical disciplines. This system has since contributed enormously to improving the standards in anesthesiology and related disciplines, and meant that Japanese anesthesiology stands almost on par with Western practice.

However, little has been reported about the fact that the origin of this qualification system, particularly the "specially approved designation" (tokushu hyobo ka) dates back to the "Board on Medical Service System" (iyakuseido chosakai) (BMSS) founded in 1938. No mention of this board and its subsequent development has made in previous articles.[1-4] Although I have described several papers on this subject, they were written in Japanese, making them inaccessible to most Western medical historians.[5,6] In this section, detailed information is provided concisely to allow better understanding of the history of the qualification system of anesthesiology in Japan.

1) The Board on Medical Service System

In July 1938, the BMSS was founded by imperial ordinance to improve medical care system in Japan. One of the topics discussed by one of the ad hoc committees of the board was the specialty designation for medical practice. This was needed because there was no qualification system for any specialty at that time in Japan, and practitioners simply claimed various specialty designations, causing confusions among patients. In December 1939, the committee decided to establish "generally (legally) approved designations" (hotei shinryo ka, or ippan shinryo ka), indicating general practice abilities, and "specially approved designations" (senmon ka), which indicated specialized abilities of practitioners. Tentatively, practitioners could also use any of the following 38 "generally (legally) approved designations" as "specially approved designations.":

Internal medicine, digestive organ disease (gastroenterological disease), respiratory disease, hemodynamic disease (circulatory disease, cardiac disease), metabolic disease, nephrologic disease, neurological disease (brain disease, cerebrospinal disease, or psychiatric disease), infectious disease, surgery, oral surgery, visceral surgery, orthopedic surgery, proctology, uro–genital disease (demimonde disease, venereal disease, or urology), dermatology, obstetrics and gynecology (obstetrics or gynecology), pediatrics, ophthalmology, otorhinolaryngology (otology, rhinology, or laryngology), radiology (roentgenology or X–ray), and physical therapy (physiotherapy) (each Japanese designation has a suffix "ka" to mean a specialty.)[7]

Practitioners could freely utilize these in signs and advertisements. Concerning the "specially approved designations," they were to be recognized in near future by the "Specialty Certification Board on Designation" (senmon hyobo shinsa i–inkai). This ad hoc committee's plan was included in the "Improvement Policy of Medical Service System (iyakuseido kaizen hosaku)" and approved by the committee. In February 1942, the "National Medical Service Law (kokumin iryo ho)" (NMSL) was promulgated, which was based mainly on the "Improvement Policy of Medical Service System." However, no records substantiate the establishment of the "Specialty Certification Board on Designation," which was probably not established because of the war.

2) The Medical Service Law

In July 1947, the government established the "Council of Medical Service System (iryo seido shingikai)" (CMSS) to revive the medical care system after the disruption of the war. The council requested the BMSS, which continued after the war, to revise the NMSL. One year later in July 1948, after discussions at meetings of the BMSS and the CMSS, the government promulgated the "Medical Service Law" (iryo ho) (MSL), which was based mainly on the NMSL of 1942. According to this new MSL, the "generally (legally) approved designations" were limited to the following 15 designations, which comprised less than 40% of the original 38 designations in the NMSL.

> Internal medicine, psychiatry, pediatrics, surgery, orthopedic surgery, dermatology, urology, obstetrics and gynecology (or obstetrics or gynecology), ophthalmology, otorhinolaryngology, and physiotherapy (or radiology).

Some practitioners, such as those who had used respiratory diseases, proctology, or venereal disease designations, fiercely opposed this new law. Furthermore, they requested that the Ministry of Health and Welfare (MHW) grant "specially approved designations," to those that were excluded, with the recommendation that the minister of the MHW be able to approve them based on Article 40, Paragraph 1, Clause 3 of the MSL. In response, the ministry founded the "Medical Ethics Council" (MEC) in November 1948 to discuss this issue. However, in March 1949, the council decided not to recognize those excluded designations as "specially approved designations," and the ministry issued a notice that further designations would not be approved.

In response to this challenge, practitioners raised stiff objections to the council and the MHW, and the Japan Medical Association (JMA) began a vigorous campaign for the approval of the removed designations by lobbying four physician representatives of the JMA. In April 1950, following designations were finally approved as "generally (legally) approved designations": digestive disease, respiratory disease, circulatory disease, neurological disease, venereal disease, and proctology. Although proctology was to be approved as "specially approved designation," the term "specially" contained a discriminative, inferior meaning, and the JMA strongly insisted proctology be included among "generally approved designations."

3) Approval of registered anesthesiologists

In 1957, three years after its foundation, the Japan Society of Anesthesiology (JAS) conducted a survey to identify the number of anesthesia practitioners and to start the recruitment of young physicians. A questionnaire was distributed to all JSA members by including it in the society's semi–official journal *Masui*. At the time, the JSA had a membership of 1100, of which 419 responded to the survey. The relatively low response of 38.1% (419/1100) can be attributed to the fact that the readership included many basic scientists who were not clinical practitioners. The collated data showed the following results: 69 physicians practiced anesthesia exclusively;

among them 30 (7.2%, 30/419) were members of anesthesiology departments at universities or medical colleges. The remaining 39 (9.3%, 39/419) were affiliated with other specialties such as surgery, orthopedics, or obstetrics. Physicians who occasionally administered anesthetics, considered part–time anesthetists, numbered 350 (83.5%, 350/419) and had various affiliations. Although the survey provides only a rough estimation, it is apparent that few full–time anesthesiologists were practicing in the early 1960s. The JAS concluded that to increase the number of full–time anesthesiologists or members of anesthesia departments at universities and medical colleges, anesthesiology must be included in the "generally approved designations" in the MSL along with internal medicine and surgery.

Despite sustained petitions by the JSA requesting the inclusion of "anesthesia" among the "generally approved designations" in the MSL, the MHW refused them because MHW was under the dominant influence of the JMA, which was presided by Taro Takemi who opposed the JSA's proposal. Professor Yamamura of the University of Tokyo, the president of the Sixth Annual Meeting of the JSA, and Associate Professor Amano of Keio University became aware that the MEC was key to the approval, with Takemi and Hiroshige Shiota being eminent members. Yamamura and Amano contacted with Takemi and Shiota to explain the status of anesthesiology and the necessity of its recognition as a medical specialty, but Takemi and Shiota had limited understanding of the difficult status of the practice of anesthesia in Japan. Yamamura, Amano, and several members of the Tokyo Society of Anesthesiologists also held institutes on anesthesia for staff members of the MHW to further the understanding of the importance of anesthesiology in clinical medicine.

After much wavering, the MEC finally approved the petition in February 1960, and anesthesiology became a "specially approved designation." This designation means that any physician who wanted to be a "registered anesthesiologist" needed specific permission from the MHW. However, the truth of the background of this approval was likely that the JMA and MHW would not evaluate anesthesiology as being par with internal medicine, surgery or other specialties, because anesthesia was still perceived to be a simple procedure that could be performed by a nurse. Indeed, the word "specially" tinged with the implication of an "inferior status."

4) Qualification of board certified anesthesiologists

Eligibility for registration as an anesthesiologist (registered anesthesiologist) could be met under one of three categories: Category (1) more than two years' exclusive practice of anesthesia at an adequate hospital under an adequate mentor; Category (2) those with more than two year's practice of anesthesia and administration of tracheal anesthesia in more than 300 patients; Category (3) those ineligible under Categories 1 or 2 but with experience in anesthesia equal to or higher than that of Categories 1 and 2. In Category 1, the definition of "an adequate mentor" became an issue for further discussion because physicians could not be eligible for Category 1, and therefore could not become registered anesthesiologists without training under an "adequate mentor" of anesthesiology.

In March 1962, after much discussion, JSA board members decided to implement the following system for board certification. First, the JSA would establish a board of examiners and select its members. Second, the examiners would conduct written, oral, and practical examinations of eligible candidates for board certification. By the end of March 1962, potential examiner candidates were selected from among professors and chairpersons of anesthesiology departments at universities and colleges, according to their curriculum vitae, academic achievements, and clinical experiences. On approval, these successful candidates became the first board certified anesthesiologists. They were Hideo Yamamura, Akira Inamoto, Ken–ichi Iwatsuki, Michinosuke Amano, Kodo Furukawa, Tetsuji Furukawa, Toshihide Yonezawa, Takeo Takahashi, and Nobuo Nishimura. Together, these anesthesiologists decided that eligibility for the board examination would depend on three conditions, that is, candidates (1) should be registered anesthesiologists, (2) should have been a JSA member for more than three consecutive years, and (3) should have more than five years' experience in exclusive practice of various methods of anesthesia. In February 1963, more than 50 candidates (the exact number remains unknown) took the first written, oral, and practical examinations, and 35 were qualified. This was the first qualification system in the history of medical practice in Japan.

Before the efforts of the Japanese Medical Specialty Board in May 2014, the JSA had started in 2013 to revise the current qualification system to include three steps: the JSA Qualified Anesthesiologists; the JSA Board Certified Anesthesiologists; and Fellows of the JSA. The JSA Qualified Anesthesiologists should complete two years' exclusive training in an anesthesia program at recognized hospital groups, and should be the registered anesthesiologists. The JSA Board Certified Anesthesiologists should be the JSA Qualified Anesthesiologists, and should experience in the following: 25 pediatric surgeries in children aged less than 6 years, 10 cesarean sections, 25 cardiovascular surgeries, 25 cases of thoracic surgery, and 25 neurosurgical procedures. They should also have completed the provider courses of American Heart Association's Advanced Cardiovascular Life Support or American Heart Association's Pediatric Advanced Life Support, and they should passed the written, oral, and practical examinations set by the JSA. In addition to these, they should obtain 50 credits: 30 credits for attendance at academic meetings and the remaining 20 credits for academic achievements. Finally, Fellows of the JSA are those who have more than 4 years of clinical experiences after becoming approved as board certified anesthesiologists and have sufficient ability to instruct board certified anesthesiologists.[8]

References and Remarks

1. Yamamura H. Advances in Anesthesiology in Japan. *Proceedings of the 17th General Meetings of the Japanese Association of Medical Sciences.* Nagoya, Japanese Medical Sciences, 1967. p.843–8.
2. Yamamura H. Past and Perspective of Anesthesiology in Our Country. *J. Japanese Society Clinical Anesthesia* 1986; 6: 1–7.
3. Yamamura H. Historical details on the emergence of registered anesthesiologists and board certified anesthesiologists in Japan. In: Fujita T. and Matsuki A. eds. *The History of Japanese Anesthesiology. Source Materials* (Vol.1). Tokyo, Kokuseido Shuppan, 1987. p.63–8.
4. Amano M. The history of modern anesthesiology in Japan (3)–35th to 51st year of the Showa–. *Rinsho Masui* 1977; 1: 228–37.
5. Matsuki A. The Background for Governmental Accreditation of "Anesthesiology" as a Specially Approved Medical Specialty (1) and (2). *Masui* 2014; 63: 594–9, 706–11.
6. Matsuki A. Several issues before and after the recognition of "Anesthesiology" as Specially Approved Specialty (1) and (2). *Masui* 2015; 64: 675–9, 780–3.
7. The Medical Affairs Bureau of the Ministry of Health and Welfare. ed. *A Hundred –Year History of the Medical Service System.* (*Document material volume*). (*Isei hyakunen shi, shiryo hen*). Tokyo, Gyosei, 1976. p.124.
8. www.anesth.or.jp// info/: managerial regulations of the qualification system (May 15, 2016)

8 Anesthesia-related Papers in the Quadrennial Meetings of the Japanese Association of Medical Sciences
 –Focusing on Professor Yamamura's presentations–

In April 2015, the Japanese Association of Medical Sciences (JAMS) celebrated its 29th general meeting in Kyoto. The history of the JAMS dates back to 1902 when its first general meeting was held in Tokyo under the title "Japanese United Association of Medical Sciences."[1] The general meeting was to be held every four years in the east (Tokyo) or the west (Osaka or Kyoto). In 1910, when the third general meeting was held in Osaka, the association was renamed to the JAMS. The reason for the exclusion of the term "United" remains unknown; however, it was likely because the term "association" itself contained the meaning of "united societies."

There was a reason that they included the term "united" in the title of "Japanese United Association of Medical Sciences" in 1902. In the end of the 19th century and beginning of the 20th century, under the influence of the German medical system, physicians of each specialty began organizing their own societies by specialty in Japan: the Japanese Association of Anatomists (the first title was the Society of Anatomy) and the Oto-Rhino-laryngological Society of Japan (the first title was the Tokyo Oto-Rhino-Laryngological Society) in 1893; the Japan Pediatric Society (the first title was the Pediatric Research Society) in 1896; the Japanese Ophthalmological Society in 1897; Japan Surgical Society in 1898; the Japanese Society of Gastroenterology (the first title was the Digestive Organ Diseases Research Society) in 1899; the Japanese Dermatological Association in 1900; the Japan Society of Obstetrics and Gynecology (the first title was the Japan Society of Gynecology) in 1901; the Japanese Society of Neurology in 1902; and the Japanese Society of Internal Medicine in 1903. Although many societies were established in the field of medicine, most physicians became aware of the necessity to discuss and exchange opinions in a joint and multidisciplinary meeting. Accordingly, the "Japanese United Association of Medical Sciences" was organized.

In 1890, before the "Japanese United Association of Medical Sciences" was founded in 1902 , there had been a society called the "Japanese Association of Medical Sciences," which was organized by the members of Itsuyukai, a private society of eminent physicians at the time.[2] The first general meeting of this society was held in Tokyo in 1890; however, lectures were only by eminent members of the association, and presentations and discussions were not allowed to practitioner members, leading to disfavor of the association by many practitioners. Although the second meeting of the association was held in 1893, the association was dissolved soon after. Thus, these two meetings were neglected in the present discussion to avoid unnecessary confusion.

During the half century between the first general meeting of the JAMS in 1902 and its 14th meeting in 1955, there was no anesthesia-related presentation. This reflected the fact that the Japanese medical world at the time had no concern about the practice of anesthesia and that no remarkable advancements that provoked the physicians' concerns were made in the field of anesthesia. Behind this, there was a generally accepted concept among physicians that the practice of anesthesia was simple procedures to be performed by nurses and not by physicians, which was not a topic to be presented and discussed at the JAMS meetings.

Professor Hideo Yamamura of the University of Tokyo was the first anesthesiologist to present a paper at the 15th general meeting of the JAMS in 1959 in Tokyo. The paper titled "The status of anesthesiology: pre-, intra-, and post-operative management of surgical patients." It was 5 years after the foundation of the JSA. This presentation is considered important in the history of anesthesia in Japan because this was the proof that physicians from various medical fields enjoyed his presentation and approved anesthesiology as one of the specialties in clinical medicine. Four years later at the 16th general meeting of the JAMS in Osaka, Yamamura was a special speaker and his lecture titled "Artificial Respiration" was one of the main topics in the specilty. At the 17th general meeting of the JAMS in Nagoya in 1967, he presented a lecture titled "The History of Anesthesia in Japan" which summarized the developing process of anesthesia beginning with Seishu Hanaoka in Japan. Thereafter, he presented the papers as one of the representatives of the JSA at the general meeting of the JAMS as follows: "Precautions Against Blood Gas Abnormality" (1971), "Clinical Aspects of Acid-Base Imbalance" (1975), and "Clinical Aspects of Pain" (1979).

He became the chairman and professor of the Department of Anesthesiology at the University of Tokyo in 1956, and retired from the position in 1980. It is noted that he was always the speaker at every general meeting of the JAMS during his 24 years' service, exemplifying that he enormously contributed to the Japanese medical science, as a representative of the JSA. No such example can be found in any other fields of medical specialties. This fact clearly proves that he is the greatest benefactor to whom Japanese anesthesiology is deeply indebted.[3]

References and Remarks

1. Committee on records of the 25th General Meeting of the Japanese Association of Medical Sciences. ed. *A Hundred–Year History of the Japanese Association of Medical Sciences*. Tokyo, The 25th General Meeting of the Japanese Association of Medical Sciences, 1999.
2. Anonym. Itsuyukai. *Tokyo Iji Shinshi* 1885; (407): 92.
3. Matsuki A. *Unknown Episodes in the history of anesthesia in Japan* (*Postwar period*). Tokyo, Shinkokoeki Ishoshuppanbu, 2014. p.247–58.

Appendix I Revised Chronology of the History of Anesthesia in Japan

This chronology describes the important and interesting events associated with the history of anesthesia in Japan. These events have been primarily obtained from monographs on the subject. This task was undertaken by the current author to provide readers a more detailed perspective of the history of anesthesia in Japan. The lunar calendar used is prior to December 3rd, 1872. An asterisk (*) indicates the event in which the month is not identified.

Pioneers in Anesthesiology–Introduction to the study of the history of anesthesiology–. Tokyo, Kokuseido Shuppan, 1983.
Chronology from Fifty Year History of the Japanese Society of Anesthesiologists. (edited by Matsuki A. et al.) *Masui* 2004; 53: S302–19.
The Roots of Anesthesiology. Tokyo, Kokuseido Shuppan, 2005
Seishu Hanaoka and Mafutsusan. Tokyo, Shinkokoeki Ishoshuppanbu, 2006.
The Origin of Anesthesiology. Tokyo, Shinkokoeki Ishoshuppanbu, 2006.
The Origin of Anesthesiology, continued. Tokyo, Shinkokoeki Ishoshuppanbu, 2009.
A New Study on the History of Anesthesiology in Japan. Tokyo, Kokuseido Shuppan, 2010.
Seishu Hanaoka and His Medicine – A Japanese Pioneer of Anesthesia and Surgery –. Hirosaki, Hirosaki University Press, 2011.
The Acceptance of Anesthesiology and Its Development of Anesthesiology in Japan. Tokyo, Shinkokoeki Ishoshuppanbu, 2011.
A Short History of Anesthesia in Japan. Hirosaki, Hirosaki University Press, 2013.
New Development in the Study of Seishu Hanaoka. Tokyo, Shinkokoeki Ishoshuppanbu, 2013.
Unknown Episodes in the History of Anesthesia in Japan (*Postwar period*). Tokyo, Shinkokoeki Ishoshuppanbu, 2014.
Unknown Episodes in the History of Anesthesia in Japan (*Prewar period*). Tokyo, Shinkokoeki Ishoshuppanbu, 2016.

Important and Interesting Events
Associated with the History of Anesthesia in Japan

733
Jun.   Okura Yamanoue introduces Hua Tuo, a great ancient Chinese physician.

1672
Aug.   Korean morning glory (*Datura alba Nees*) is cultivated in Edo (Tokyo).

1686
May   Poppies are cultivated in the Tsugaru district (The most northern part of mainland Japan) for producing opium.

1689
Nov.   Tokumei Takamine of Ryukyu successfully treats the cleft lip of Shoeki (a grandson of the King Shotei); however, Takamine does not use general anesthetic.

1746
Mar.   Hoyoku Takashi publishes *Honetsugi Ryoji Chohoki*, mentioning several anesthetics including *Seikotsu Mayaku* (*Anesthetics for bone setting*).

1782
*   Seishu Hanaoka visits Kyoto to study medicine and surgery. Sadakichi Iwanaga is one of the preceptors of surgery.

1785
Feb.   Seishu Hanaoka returns to his homeland Hirayama after 3 years of training.

1795
May   Seishu Hanaoka revisits Kyoto to study Dutch style ointments.

1796
May   Shutei Nakagawa describes in *Mayaku Ko* that Hanaoka is

successful in producing types of general anesthesia using on more than 10 human volunteers.

1804
Oct.13   Seishu Hanaoka administers the general anesthetic *Mafutsusan* to 60–year–old Kan Aiya for excising a breast cancer tumor. This is the first recorded case of general anesthesia in the world.

1805
Feb.23   Kan Aiya dies.

1807
Dec.   Genka Ninomiya publishes *Seikotsu Han*, mentioning an anesthetic *Seikotsu Mayaku*.

1808
Dec.   Bunken Kagami publishes *Seikotsu Shinsho*, mentioning an anesthetic *Masuisan*.

1810
*   Juntatsu Miyakawa from Kanazawa Feudal Province performs breast cancer tumor excisions on 2 or more patients using *Mafutsusan* in Edo (Tokyo) by this year.

1813
Oct.   Ryukei Sugita performs an excision of a breast cancer tumor under general anesthesia using *Mafutsusan* in Edo, and publishes a brochure entitled *Ryo Nyugan Ki* to describe the case.

1827
May   Franz von Siebold of the Dutch Factory in Nagasaki removes a boy's head wen (10 cm in diameter) without anesthesia. He administers opium to the boy for relieving postoperative pain. The boy develops a coma and dies on the seventh day after surgery.

1835
Oct. 2   Seishu Hanaoka dies.

1840
* Gendai Kamata publishes *Geka Kihai Zufu*, including several illustrations of patients under general anesthesia.

1847
Nov. Gencho Honma publishes *Yoka Hiroku* in 10 volumes.

1848
Aug. Otto Mohnike informs Soken Narabayashi of chloroform analgesia in Nagasaki.

1850
Mar. Seikei Sugita translates J. Schlesinger's Dutch monograph on ether anesthesia and titles it *Ateru Kyuho Shisetsu*. Sugita coins the Japanese word "*Masui*," meaning "anesthesia" or "general anesthesia."

1851
Aug. Otto Mohnike informs Shinsuke Maeda of the ineffectiveness of ether inhalation for surgical operation in Nagasaki.

* Gendai Kamata publishes *Geka Kihai* in 10 volumes.

1855
* Seikei Sugita is unsuccessful in producing general anesthesia using ether in a burn scar patient and a breast cancer patient. The agent is prepared by Ryuho Shima.

1857
Apr. Gencho Honma amputates the right lower extremity of a male patient above the knee joint using *Mafutsusan*. This is the first amputation above the knee joint in Japan.

1858
Dec. Gonsai Miyake reproduces Benjamin Hobson's *First Lines of the Practice of Surgery in the West* (1857) as *Sei–i Ryakuron*, in which chloroform anesthesia is described.

1859
  Jan.   Gencho Honma publishes *Zoku Yoka Hiroku* in five volumes.

1860
  May   Japanese physicians Ryugen Miyazaki and Domin Kawasaki, and surgeon Hakugen Murayama, observe William T. G. Morton administer ether anesthesia at The Gross Clinic in Philadelphia.

  *   Keisaku Ninomiya instructs Shoan Shinoda regarding the preparation of chloroform.

1861
  Jun.   Gemboku Ito administers chloroform anesthesia to Yoshijiro Sakuragawa before amputating his right foot. This is the first recorded chloroform anesthesia in Japan.

1862
  Feb.   Ryoan Imamura discloses the prescription of *Maftsusan* in *Ijikeigen*.

1863
  Jul.   Shinryo Tsuboi translates a Dutch book on ether anesthesia and entitles *Ateru Kyuho Shiken Setsu*. The original book remains unknown.

1868
  Jan.   William Willis administers chloroform anesthesia to treat soldiers wounded in the Toba and Fushimi Battles.

  Jan.   Kenzo Yoshida, who had observed Willis' use of chloroform, successfully administers chloroform for an abdominal operation in a male patient in Kyoto.

  Apr. ~ May   Gen-yu Hirota administers chloroform anesthesia to several wounded soldiers at Mibu, Tochigi and later in Edo.

1869
  May   Ryoun Takamatsu is thought to have used chloroform anesthesia to treat wounded soldiers from the Hakodate Battle.

1876
  Nov. Tadanori Ishiguro coins the phrases of *Kyokusho Masui* (local anesthesia) and *Zenshin Masui* (general anesthesia), and defines these terms.

1884
  *   Kinnojo Ume of the University of Tokyo arranges to import cocaine.

1884
  Apr. Tetsuya Inou–e describes the first use of cocaine in ophthalmic surgery.

1887
  Nov. Susumu Sato advocates the use of cocaine instead of chloroform anesthesia.

1890
  Apr. Susumu Sato presents a paper on local anesthesia with cocaine at the first meeting of the Japan Medical Association.

1893
  Apr. Waichiro Okada presents a paper on local anesthesia using cocaine and Keizo Dohi reads a paper on anesthetic method at the second meeting of the Japan Medical Association. (This association is disbanded.)

1896
  Mar. Quincke's spinal puncture is introduced to Japan.

1897
  Mar. The 50th Anniversary of Morton's Public demonstration of ether anesthesia is conducted at Ueno, Tokyo.

1898
  Apr. The Japan Surgical Society (JSS) is founded.

1899
  Jan. Orio Terada translates Carl Schleich's *Schmerzlose Operationen*

and publishes it under the title *Mutsu Shujutsu*.

Apr. The First Annual Meeting of the JSS is conducted. Sankichi Sato is the first president.

1901
* Otojiro Kitagawa, Ryohei Azuma, and Hayazo Ito administer spinal anesthesia using cocaine and eucaine independently. Kitagawa administers spinal morphine for pain relief in two patients. He is one of the first to administer spinal morphine for alleviating intractable pain in the world.

1903
Aug. Jun-ichiro Watanabe introduces Jacoby's line to Japan. (This is an imaginary line across the highest points of the both iliac crests).

1906
* Tsugushige Kondo imports an anesthetic machine from Germany (possibly Wohlgemuth's apparatus).

1911
May Yoshihiro Miwa publishes *Local Anesthesia* (*Kyokusho masui*).

1912
Mar. Yutaka Tongu publishes *Sacral and Lumbar Anesthesia* (*Senkotsu oyobi yozui masuiho*).

Apr. Shigeki Nakayama reads his special report on general anesthesia and Nobushiro Ueno reads his paper on local anesthesia at the 12th Annual Meeting of the JSS. These are the first special presentations on anesthesia at the JSS meeting.

May Yuta Hosoya and Jugyo Nagano translate Heinrich Braun's *Die Lokalanästhesie* and publish it under the title *Kinsei Kyokusho Masui*.

May First law suit concerning death during chloroform anesthesia occurs. The plaintiff's claim is rejected. (The accident occurred on June 8, 1911, and the surgeon was sued this year.)

1913
- Dec. Gonpei Matsui reports a case of death during ether anesthesia. Death is considered to have been caused by status thymico-lymphaticus. This is the first reported case of status thymico-lymphaticus as a cause of anesthetic death in Japan.

1915
- Jan. Yutaka Tongu publishes *Conduction Anesthesia* (*Dentatsu masuiho*).

1916
- Jan. Keijiro Kitamura publishes *Methods of Local Anesthesia* (*Kyokusho mahiho*).

- Mar. Yoshihiro Miwa publishes *General Therapeutics, General Anesthesia, Local Anesthesia, Anti–sepsis and Asepsis*. This book is considered to be the first comprehensive textbook on the introduction to anesthesia in Japan.

1921
- May Koshiro Nakagawa uses ethyl alcohol intravenously to produce general anesthesia. (*Tohoku J. Exp. Med*. 1921; 2: 81–126.)

1923
- Sep. Seigo Minami reports three cases of crush syndrome. This is the first report of the syndrome in the world. (*Virch. Arch. Path. Anat*. 1923; 245: 247–67.)

1924
- Apr. A report is presented from the First Department of Surgery at Kyushu University, mentioning higher postoperative mortality in patients who received general anesthesia than in those who received local anesthesia.

1925
- Apr. A debate on thoracotomy begins between Professor Torikata of Kyoto University and Professor Sekiguchi of Tohoku University. This debate continues until 1938.

- Apr. First reported death caused by spinal anesthesia. The patient dies on April 27, four days after surgery.

Nov. Takeshi Abe publishes *New Local Anesthesia* (*Shinsen Kyokusho Masui*).

1933
  Mar. Hayao Nakatani visits the Mayo Clinic and advocates American anesthesiology.

1935
  Jan. Masataka Maeda elucidates a mechanism of excitement during anesthetic induction with ether inhalation. Later, he confirms that the same mechanism is acting during the administration of chloroform.

1936
  Apr. Daisuke Nagae studies anesthesiology at the Mayo Clinic under John S. Lundy and Franc C. Mann. Nagae is a military attaché at the Japanese Embassy in Washington, D.C.

1937
  Nov. Daisuke Nagae meets Kenji Tanaka at the Johns Hopkins Hospital in Baltimore. Both are aware of the importance of general anesthesia.

1938
  Dec. Daisuke Nagae introduces tracheal anesthesia using an illustration of a tracheal tube to Japan.

1940
  Mar. Kentaro Shimizu visits Percival S. Bailey's department at the University of Illinois as a research fellow.

  May Park Rang–Su reads a paper on spinal anesthesia with hyperbaric solution with 10% glucose at the annual meeting of the JSS.

1941
  Aug. Makoto Saito and Park Rang–Su describe their paper about spinal anesthesia using a hyperbaric solution with 10% glucose. They

propose the saddle block technique.

1942
Oct.   Reizo Takashima publishes *Anesthetic Method* (*Masuiho*).

1949
Jan.   Makoto Saito publishes *Local Anesthesia and General Anesthesia* (*Kyokusho masuiho oyobi zenshin masuiho*).

1950
Feb.   Yoshio Kusama of Keio University meets Crawford F. Sams, a brigadier general of GHQ, requesting for a medical mission to Japan.

Mar.   Sams requests the Unitarian Service Committee to send a medical mission.

Jul.4   Seiji Kimoto and his colleagues of the Second Department of Surgery at the University of Tokyo perform a mastectomy under tracheal anesthesia (ether) using a Japanese anesthetic machine. This is the first recorded tracheal anesthesia in Japan. The patient is a 50–year–old woman named Yasu Kawanishi. Shuichi Hayashi and Tetsu Watanuki administer the anesthesia.

Jul.12   Kentaro Shimizu of the First Department at the University of Tokyo returns to Japan from his second visit to the United States.

Jul.18   Kentaro Shimizu emphasizes the importance of anesthesiology at a round–table discussion hosted by the editorial board of the Journal *Geka*.

Jul.19   Meyer Saklad delivers lectures on anesthesiology at the Japanese–American Joint Conference on Medical Education (JAJCME) in Tokyo. Kentaro Shimizu is the translator.

Jul. 20   Shuichi Hayashi presents his paper on two cases of tracheal anesthesia at a meeting of Surgical Treatment of Pulmonary Tuberculosis in Sendai.

Jul. 24   The JAJCME formally commences. Several members arrive behind schedule because of the Korean War.

Jul.   Michinosuke Amano of Keio University visits the United States as a student of the Government Appropriation for Relief in an Occupied Area and studies anesthesiology at the University of Chicago.

Sep.   An anesthesia group is formed on Professor Shimizu's order at the First Department of Surgery at the University of Tokyo. Hideo Yamamura is the chief.

Oct.   A Heidbrink "midget–type" anesthetic machine is purchased by Keio University.

Oct.   The clinical use of thiopental begins at the Second Department of Surgery at the University o Tokyo.

Nov.   Hideo Yamamura reads a paper on anesthesia at the 492nd Meeting of the Tokyo Surgical Society and asserts that he must be an anesthesiologist, instead of a surgeon.

Nov.   Tokuji Ichikawa et al publish *Surgical Operations and Anesthesia* (*Shujutsu to masui*).

*   Nitrous oxide is marketed

1951

Jan.   Wasaburo Maeda edits and publishes *The Most Recent Surgery and Anesthsia* (*Mottomo atarashii geka to masui*). This is the proceedings of the lectures by Professor Paul W. Shafer and Dr. Meyer Saklad at the JAJCME.

Jan.   Fumiyoshi Iida and colleagues report the first clinical use of thiopental.

Apr.   Wasaburo Maeda delivers the presidential address "We are in dire need of education and research in anesthesiology." at the 51st Annual Meeting of the JSS.

May ~Jun.	Perry P. Volpitto delivers lectures at Tohoku University, Keio University, and Kyushu University. He is a member of the Second Medical Mission of the Unitarian Service Committee.
Dec.	Tamotsu Fukuda et al publish *The Most Recent Anesthesia* (*Saishin masuigaku*).
*	Japanese gas machines are marketed by Ichikawa Shiseido.
*	Cyclopropane is marketed.

1952

Jan.	Domestic thiopental is marketed.
Apr.	A journal entitled *Masui* is published from Kokuseido Shuppan.
Apr.	Hideo Yamamura describes the first clinical use of thiamylal sodium.
Jun.	Naoyuki Hoshiko and Ken-ichi Iwatsuki publish *New Introduction to Anesthesia* (*Atarashii masuigaku nyumon*).
Jul. 16	The Independent Department of Anesthesiology is established at the University of Tokyo. Associate professor Hideo Yamamura is the chief.
Jul.17	The First *Anesthesia Conference* was conducted by Wasaburo Maeda at Keio University.
Jul.18	The *Joint Research Group on Anesthesia* supported by the Ministry of Education is initiated. The chairman is Masao Muto of Tohoku University and 22 members from various other universities join the research group.
Jul.	Hideo Itokawa, Kentaro Shimizu et al. use an electroencephalograph during ether and thiopental anesthesia.
Aug.	Michinosuke Amano hosts the *Institute on Anesthesia* at Keio

University, sponsored by the Keio Medical Association. Nineteen institutes are conducted until the end of 1954 at various sites.

Nov.   d–Tubocurarine is marketed.

1953

May   Michinosuke Amano publishes *Anesthesiology* (*Masuigaku*).

Jun.   Tetsu Watanuki publishes *Endotracheal Anesthesia and Its Precautions* (*Kikan–nai masuiho oyobi sono chuiten*).

Oct.   A promotors' meeting is conducted to discuss the founding of the Tokyo Society of Anesthesiologists. The members are Seizo Iwai, Shigeru Kawata, Mitsuko Nakamura, Shoji Okawa, Shigeru Shiozawa, Yoshitane Watabe, and Toru Yamamoto.

Nov.   The first general meeting of the Tokyo Society of Anesthesiology is conducted. There are initially 23 members.

1954

Jan.   Kingo Shinoi, Kentaro Shimizu, Tamotsu Fukuda, Seiji Kimoto, Wasaburo Maeda, Masao Muto, Hideo Yamamura, and Michinosuke Amano conduct a meeting to discuss founding an anesthesia society at the Japanese restaurant Orizuru.

Apr. 30   The foundation of the *Japan Society of Anesthesiology* (JSA) is approved at the council meeting of the JSS.

May   The JSA is founded.

May   Hideo Yamamura publishes *Clinical Anesthesiology* (*Rinsho masuigaku*).

May   Shinobu Miyamoto publishes *A Practice of Inhalation Anesthesia* (*Kyunyu masui no jissai*).

Jun.   The first meeting of the Tokai Anesthesia Research Society is conducted in Nagoya.

Oct. The first Annual Meeting of the JSA is conducted in Tokyo. Masao Muto is the president.

Oct. *Masui* is the semi–official journal of the JSA (since Vol.3 No.4).

1955
Mar.14 *Colloquium on Anesthesia* suggested by Michinosuke Amano is conducted. It is disbanded by September 1961 to develop the Meetings of the Kanto Regional Society of the JSA.

Oct. Yutaka Onchi publishes *Reconsideration of Anesthesia* (*Masui no hansei*).

Nov. Akira Horita of the University of Washington School of Medicine publishes a paper in *Anesthesiology*. He is the first Japanese to publish a paper in *Anesthesiology*.

* Suxamethonium (succinylcholine chloride) is marketed.

1956
Apr. Joseph F. Artusio, Jr. delivers lectures at the Symposia on Anesthesiology conducted at the University of Tokyo, Keio University, Kyoto University and other universities. He is a member of the Third Medical Mission of the Unitarian Service Committee.

Aug. F. C. Dye and V. L. Traina of the 6110th United States Air Force Hospital at Nagoya publish *The Far East Journal of Anesthesia* in Nagoya. (discontinued in August 1966 with the last issue of Vol.5 No.3.)

1957
Feb. The JSA conducts a membership survey using a questionnaire as a survey instrument. Only 30 (7.2%) members exclusively practice anesthesia.

May The first *Nitrous Oxide Seminar* is conducted at Nagaoka, Niigata Prefecture (disbanded in 1965).

Jun.	The JSA is approved as the 45th member of the Japanese Association of Medical Sciences.

1958

Mar.	Akira Inamoto of Kyoto University initiates the clinical use of halothane.
Nov.	The Tokyo Society of Anesthesiologists is founded.
*	Kingo Shinoi of Tokyo Medical College, the president of the 5th Annual Meeting of the JSA, submits a written document to the Ministry of Health and Welfare petitioning the approval of anesthesiology as a designated specialty.

1959

Jan.	Hideo Yamamura, the president of the 6th Annual Meeting of the JSA initiates a signature–collecting campaign for approval of anesthesiology as a designated specialty.
Jan.14	The JSA and the Tokyo Society of Anesthesiologists conduct a seminar on anesthesia for 9 members of the Ministry of Health and Welfare.
Jan.16	Anesthesiology is provisionally accredited as a "specially approved specialty" by the Medical Ethics Council.
Apr.	Hideo Yamamura presents a paper at the 15th General Meeting of the Japanese Association of Medical Sciences in Tokyo. He is the first anesthesiologist to present a paper at the association.
Apr.	The JSA and the Tokyo Society of Anesthesiologists conduct the second seminar on anesthesia for 10 members of the Ministry of Health and Welfare.
Oct.	Halothane is marketed.
*	Hideo Yamamura, the president of the 6th Annual Meeting of the JSA, resubmits a document to the Ministry of Health and Welfare requesting approval of anesthesiology as a designation.

1960

Feb. Anesthesiology is formally accredited as a "specially approved designation" for medical care by the Medical Ethics Council.

Apr. The qualification committee on registered anesthesiologists is organized. Akira Inamoto, Ken-ichi Iwatsuki, Michinosuke Amano, Hideo Yamamura, and Kumio Yamashita are members.

Jun. The first meeting of the Tohoku Regional Society of Anesthesiology of the JSA is conducted in Sendai. The president is Ken-ichi Iwatsuki.

Sep. The JSA is recognized as a member of the World Federation of Societies of Anaesthesiologists.

Dec. The First Meeting of the Kansai Regional Society of Anesthesiology of the JSA is held in Kyoto. The president is Akira Inamoto.

* Hexocarbacholine and carbolonium are marketed.

1961

Jun. The First Meeting of the Tokai Regional Society of the JSA is conducted. The president remains unknown.

Jul. The Society for Painless Delivery (*Mutsubunben Kenkyukai*) is established. (The society develops to the Japan Society for Obstetric Anesthesia and Perinatology in 2008.)

Aug. A journal *Delivery and Anesthesia* is published.

Oct. The First Meeting of the Kanto Regional Society of the JSA is conducted at Juntendo University. The president is Hideo Yamamura.

1962

Mar. The Committee on Board Qualification is established. Hideo Yamamura, Akira Inamoto, Ken-ichi Iwatsuki, Michinosuke Amano, Kodo Furukawa, Tetsuji Furukawa, Toshihide Yonezawa, Takeo Takahashi, and Nobuo Nishimura are the board members.

Jul.	The Journal of Tokai Society of Anesthesiology titled *Mutsu to Masui* is issued. This is the first journal of the regional society; however it is discontinued in 1968.
Aug.	Hideo Yamamura founds the Pain Clinic at the University of Tokyo Hospital.

1963

Feb.	The first written and oral board examinations are conducted at the University of Tokyo. Practical examination is subsequently conducted at the candidates' respective hospitals. 35 candidate members are passed. Nine board examiners and 35 examinees are recognized as board qualified anesthesiologists.
Feb.	The JSA recognizes certified training hospitals in which a board qualified anesthesiologist works as the full–time specialist.
Sep.	An Exhibition of *Modern Anesthesia* is conducted at Mitsukoshi Department Store in Tokyo.
Oct.	The first meeting of the Kyushu Society of Anesthesiology in Kurume. (The president is Tetsuji Furukawa.)
*	Methoxyflurane is marketed.

1964

Nov.	The first meeting of the Chugoku Shikoku Regional Society of the JSA is conducted in Okayama. The president is undecided.

1965

*	Alcuronium is marketed.

1966

Sep.	The 2nd Asian Australasian Congress of Anaesthesiologits is conducted in Tokyo. Hideo Yamamura is the president.
Nov.	The first meeting of Hokuriku Regional Society of Anesthesiology is conducted in Kanazawa. The president is Fumio Akasu.

1967
- Jul. The clinical use of Gamma Hydroxybutylate is initiated.

- * Gallamine is marketed.

1969
- Jan. The Kyoto International Conference Center in Kyoto is selected as the venue of the 5th World Congress of Anaesthesiologists (WCA).

- Jun. The first JSA annual report is issued.

- Jul. The JSA presents commemorative shields to the following for contribution to the society: Chikashi Suzuki, Kenji Honda, Hiroshi Okamura, Eikichi Hosoya, Shuichi Hayashi, Shinobu Miyamoto, Masatoshi Takahashi, Tetsu Watanuki, Sichiro Ishikawa, Yoshio Hashimoto, Chuzo Nagaishi, Yoshiaki Takeda, Suketaro Jitsukawa, and Hiroshi Miyake.

- Aug. The Research Society of the Pain Clinic is founded. The society develops to the Japan Society of Pain Clinicians in 1985.

- Aug. A movie *Masui* (*Anesthesia*) by the JSA is produced.

- Sep. Seminar on *Anesthesia and Reanimation* is initiated. The seminar is disbanded in 1993.

- Nov. Bupivacaine is marketed.

- * Alcuronium is marketed.

1970
- Aug. A movie *Kyokusho Masui* (*local anesthesia*) is produced by Yoshitomi Pharmaceutical Co.

- * Hideo Yamamura is the editor of *Anesthesia and Neurophysiology* (International Anesthesiology Clinic Vol.8. No.1, Little Brown). He is the first Japanese to edit English monographs.

1971

Jun. Oyama and Matsuki begin the clinical use of enflurane anesthesia.

Jul. The First Hokkaido Regional Society of Anesthesiology of the JSA is conducted in Sapporo. The president is Takeo Takahashi.

* The Research Society for Pediatric Anesthesia (*Shonimasui kenkyukai*) is founded by Seizo Iwai. The society develops to the Japanese Society of Pediatric Anesthesiology in 1995.

1972

Feb. Droperidol and fentanyl are marketed.

Sep. The 5th WCA is conducted in Kyoto in the presence of the Crown Prince Akihito and Crown Princess Michiko. Hideo Yamamura is the president. Tomio Ogata delivers a special lecture on Seishu Hanaoka.

1973

Jun. Tsutomu Oyama publishes *Anesthetic Management of Endocrine Disease* from Springer. This is the first English monograph written by a single Japanese author.

* Pancuronium is marketed.

1974

Apr. Takuo Aoyagi delivers his paper on the principle of pulse-oximeter at the 13th Annual Meeting of the Japanese Medical Electronics in Osaka.

1977

Apr. The journal *Rinsho Masui* (*Clinical Anesthesia*) is published.

1979

May The emblem of the JSA, featuring a flower of datura, is decided. It is designed by the Department of Industrial Design at the Chiba University School of Engineering.

Oct. The First Korean–Japanese Joint Symposium is conducted in

Seoul.

1980
Jun.   The journal *Pain Clinic* is published.

1981
May   The JSA Prize (Yamamura Prize) is instituted.

1981
Nov.   The *journal of the Japan Society for Clinical Anesthesia* is published.

*   Enflurane is marketed.

1982
Sep.   The Japanese Society of Reanimatology is founded.

1983
Apr.   Kazuyuki Ikeda initiates clinical testing of sevoflurane.

May   Clinical testing of isoflurane begins.

Jun.   The JSA publishes *Anesthesia Terminology* (1st edition).

1985
Jun.   *Japanese Anesthesia Journals' Review* is published by VNU Science Press, the Netherlands. The Editor–in–Chief is Tsutomu Oyama. (It is discontinued in 1991 with the last issue of Vol 4. No3/4.)

1986
Jul.   The title of the JSA's official journal is decided to be the *Journal of Anesthesia*.

1987
Mar.   The official journal of the JSA, the *Journal of Anesthesia* is published.

1988
Aug.   Vecuronium is marketed.

Sep.   The Japan Society of Local Anesthesia is founded. It is disbanded in 2007.

Dec.   The Japan Society for Geriatric Anesthesia is founded.

1990
Jan.   Isoflurane and sevoflurane are marketed.

1993
Jul.   The first *Newsletter* of the JSA is issued.

Aug.   The JSA publishes *Anesthesia Terminology* (2nd revised edition).

1994
Apr.   The *Journal of the Japan Society of Pain Clinicians* is published.

1995
Apr.   The JSA Research Incentive Prize is instituted.

1998
Apr.   The JSA Social Prize is instituted.

May   The journal *Cardiovascular Anesthesia* is published.

1998
Apr.   An ad hoc committee on the incorporation of the JSA is organized.

1999
Jun.   The new terminology *Masuikagaku* proposed by A. Matsuki is adopted instead of *Masuigaku*.

2000
Jul.   October 13th is proposed to be *Anesthesia Day* by A. Matsuki.

2001
Jun.   The appellation of the society is changed from the *Japan Society of Anesthesiology* to the *Japanese Society of Anesthesiologists*. The Japanese title of the society is *Nihon Masuika Gakkai*.

Jun.   The JSA is incorporated and authorized by the government of

Japan.

2002
Apr.   The JSA publishes the third revised edition of *Anesthesia Terminology.*

2003
May   The ceremony of the 50th Annual Meeting of the JSA is conducted in Tokyo.

May   The JSA presents certificates of commendation to the following for contribution to the founding of the society: Michinosuke Amano, Ken–ichi Iwatsuki, the late Mitsuo Sato, Takeo Takahashi, Hideo Yamamura, and the the late Toshihide Yonezawa at the 50th Annual Meeting of the JSA.

2004
May   The JSA Seishu Prize is instituted.

Jun.   The commemorative issue of the 50th Annual Meeting of the JSA is published as a supplement of the journal *Masui* (Vol. 53).

2005
Dec.   The 8th Biennial Congress of the Asian and Oceanic Society of Regional Anesthesia is conducted in Chiba. The president is Kazuo Hanaoka.

2007
Jan.   Hironori Ishihara publishes *Fluid Volume Monitoring with Glucose Dilution* from Springer. This is the second English monograph by a single Japanese author.

Oct.   Rocuronium is marketed.

2008
Sep.   The JSA office is relocated from Tokyo to Kobe.

2009
May   The JSA's annual meeting is postponed to August because of the

	prevalence of a new type of influenza.
Aug.	The *Archives of the JSA* commences at the JSA office building in Kobe.
Aug.	The JSA Matsuki Prize is instituted.

2010
Jan.	The *Journal of Anesthesia* is published bimonthly.
Jun.	The 13th *Asian and Australasian Congress of Anaesthesiologists* is conducted in Fukuoka. The president is Koji Sumikawa.

2011
Mar.	Akitomo Matsuki publishes *Seishu Hanaoka and His Medicine*.
Apr.	The JSA is approved as a public service corporation.
May	The *Japanese Museum of Anesthesiology* (JMA) is established from the *JSA Archives*.
Jul.	Desflurane is marketed.

2012
Oct.	Akitomo Matsuki publishes *A Short History of Anesthesia in Japan*.

2013
Oct.	The JSA begins the revision of the current qualification system to include Qualified Anesthesiologists, Board Certified Anesthesiologists, and Fellows.

2014
Apr.	The Japanese Society of Regional Anesthesia is established.

2015
Oct.	The Japanese Anesthesia History Association is established.
Nov.	The *Journal of Anesthesia Clinical Report* (*online*) is published.

Appendix II History of Anesthesia in the United States, Great Britain, and Other Countries

Elemér K. Zsigmond (1930–2012) was a professor of anesthesiology at the Department of Anesthesiology, University of Michigan School of Medicine, Ann Arbor, Michigan, when I visited his department as a research fellow in 1972. He asked me to conduct several clinical studies on the adrenocortical responses to surgical interventions during various types of general anesthesia. Although I found these clinical investigations challenging, I asked him to allow me to conduct a private research on the history of anesthesia in the United States. I thought it essential and mandatory to conduct these historical studies to understand the background of our specialty, particularly in the United States where the first public demonstration of ether anesthesia was performed by William T. G. Morton in 1846. I was also confident that a historical approach was one of the best means for better appreciating the specialty because I had commenced my historical study of medicine in 1961 as a medical student and had a reasonable understanding of the history of medicine. Although Professor Zsigmond was not an expert on the history of anesthesiology, he generously permitted me to conduct my research on the subject and gave me several invaluable suggestions and comments.

I devoted myself to searching the shelves of medical journals in the Taubman Health Sciences Library of the medical school of the university after 6 o'clock in the afternoon on weekdays and from 9 o'clock on most Saturday mornings. The fruits of my laborious work were the writings of 10 papers on the history of anesthesia in the United States and allied countries before I left the United States in mid–December 1972. All of these studies appeared in anesthesia journals in 1973 and 1974, as shown in Appendix II. I believe several of them contributed to some extent to the progress in the historical study of the specialty in the United States, Great Britain, and other countries.

I was extremely concerned with the introduction of ether anesthesia to Great Britain because it represents a classic example of the spread of medical information, and I found that Dr. James Robinson, an American dentist in London, played an important role in the first trial of ether anesthesia in London; however, his contribution was not significantly recognized before

I referred to him. In addition to this, I found that the first British article on the discovery of ether anesthesia appeared in the *London Medical Gazette* in 1846, which was neglected in the monographs by Duncum[1] and Sykes[2] who were authorities in the field. These circumstances are described in the second and third papers reproduced in Appendix II.[3,4]

These two papers stimulated medical historians in the British isles, among them, Richard H. Ellis (1937–1995), a consultant anesthetist of St. Barthoromew Hospital, London. He was greatly stimulated by these two papers by us and was motivated to commence a study of the very early history of ether anesthesia in London because he thought that British historians, no foreign historians, should resolve unknown issues on the subjects. Thus, his two papers on the subject appeared in 1976 and 1977, 3 years after our papers.[5,6] They were his first papers on the history of the introduction of ether anesthesia to London. He confided in me this "folded" story on an excursion boat on the Thames in July 1987 when the Second International Symposium on the History of Anaesthesia was held in London and concluded our conversation by saying "I would never have begun my study on the history of anesthesia without your papers." He delivered a special presentation titled "Dr John Snow. His London residence, and the site for a commemorative plaque in London" at the opening ceremony of the symposium.[7] In subsequent years, he was very active in the study of British history of anesthesia, by reproducing classical books by John Snow[8,9] and by James Robinson.[10]

The details of complicated historical events were clarified by his substantial efforts concerning the introduction process of ether anesthesia from Boston to London at the end of 1846. I am satisfied only with the fact that our papers were a stimulus for Dr. Ellis' study on the subject, resulting in an indirect contribution of the very early history of anesthesia in London.

I edited this Appendix II in memory of Professor Elemér K. Zsigmond who graciously allowed me the opportunity to conduct my historical study, and reproduced as they were.

References

1. Duncum BM. *The Development of Inhalation Anaesthesia*. London, New York, Toronto, Oxford University Press, 1947. p.130–66.
2. Sykes WS. *Essays on the First Hundred Years of Anaesthesia* (Vol.1). Edinburgh, E.&S. Livingstone, 1960. p.48–76.
3. Matsuki A and Zsigmond EK. The First Three Days in the History of Surgical

Anaesthesia in England. *Anaesthesia* 1973; 28: 176–8.
4. Matsuki A and Zsigmond EK. The First Published Report of Morton's Ether Anaesthesia in the British Isles. *Anaesthetist* 1973; 22: 389–92.
5. Ellis RH. The Introduction of ether anaesthesia. 1. How the news was carried from Boston, Massachusetts to Gower Street, London. *Anaesthesia* 1976; 31: 766–77.
6. Ellis RH. The Introduction of ether anaesthesia to Great Britain. 2. A biographical sketch of Dr. Francis Boott. *Anaesthesia* 1977; 32: 197–208.
7. Ellis RH. Dr John Snow. His London residence, and the site for a commemorative plaque in London. In: Atkinson RS and Boulton TB. eds. *The History of Anaesthesia. Proceedings of the Second International Symposium on the History of Anaesthesia.* London, New York, Royal Society of Medicine Services, 1989. p.1–7.
8. Snow J. (a reproduction with an introductory essay by RH Ellis). *On narcotism by the inhalation of vapours.* London, New York, Royal Society of Medicine Services, 1991.
9. Ellis RH. *The case books of Jhon Snow. Med His Suppl.* 1995; i – vii: 1–633.
10. Robinson J. *A Treatise on The Inhalation of The Vapour of Ether.* (reproduced by Richard H. Ellis). London, Ballière Tindall, 1983.

1 A Census of Copies of the Original Edition of John Snow's "On the Inhalation of the Vapour of Ether in Surgical Operations"

Matsuki A and McIntyre JWR
*Proceedings of the Fourth International Symposium
on the History of Anaesthesia*
Luebeck, Draeger Druck, 1998. p.797–803.

A bibliographical survey has been profoundly made on several invaluable medical classics. In 1984, Horowitz and Collins tried a worldwide census of the original edition of Andreas Vesalius' *De humani corporis fabrica* published in 1543 to report that 154 original copies have been preserved in the world.[1] In 1988, Whitteridge and English revised Geoffrey Keynes' *Bibliography of the Writings of Dr. William Harvey* to describe in detail that seventy original copies of the first edition of so-called *De Motu Cordis* published in 1628 are existing.[2] In the field of anesthesiology, John Snow's

Table 1 Reproductions of the Original Edition of John Snow's
On the Inhalation of the Vapour of Ether in Surgical Operations

	Editor	Year	Publisher
1	Boston Medical Library	undated	Unknown, Boston, U.S.A.?
2	Wood Library–Museum with foreword by the board of the trustees	1959	Lea & Febiger, Philadelphia, U.S.A.
3	Ole Secker (This is a reproduction of the reproduced copy by the Wood Library–Museum)	1985	Janssen Pharma A/S, Birkerod, Denmark
4	Matsuki A with foreword in English and Japanese	1987	Iwanami Book Service Center, Tokyo, Japan

1 A Census of Copies of the Original Edition of John Snow's "On the Inhalation of the Vapour of Ether in Surgical Operations" 217

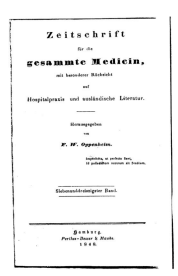

Figure 1 Autograph by John Snow on the Half title page of Matsuki's Copy

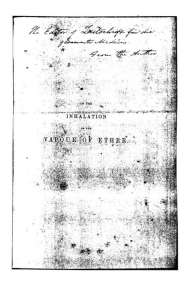

Figure 2 Title page of *Zeitschrift für gesamte Medicin*, in which Oppenheim reviewed Snow's book

first monograph entitled with *On the Inhalation of the Vapour of Ether in Surgical Operations*[3] is the most brilliant classics as evidenced by repeated reproductions for these fifty years as shown in Table 1.

When the Wood Library–Museum of Anesthesiology of the United States reproduced the book by John Snow in 1958, Professor Vincent Collins was in charge of this work and he made a census for the original edition. On our request, he wrote us on this item as follows:

> When I was secretary of the board of Directions of the Wood Library–Museum of Anesthesia, I tried in 1957–58, to determine how many copies were extant. It was believed that by the rare book dealers and Drs Macintosh and Magill there were just six copies known. They are: 1) One in the London Meidical Library (now in the Welcome Institute), 2) one at Oxford University, 3) One in the Wood Library–Museum, 4) One in the National Library of Medicine, 5) one in Yale University, Cushing Collection, and 6) One in the private collection in the United States (not identified)

When the World Congress of Anaesthesiology was held in Hamburg in

1980, I purchased by chance the original copy (Figure 1). The copy was autographed by John Snow to present to Mr Oppenheim, the editor of *Zeitschrift für gesamte Medicin* (Figure 2). Therefore, the copy possessed by (Matsuki A) is the seventh. However, no detailed bibliographical investigation has been tried on the original copies of the first edition of Snow's book on ether anesthesia published in 1847. Thus we made an international census on the book.

Method

We set out to examine the likely possession of the original copy in the United States, Canada, the United Kingdom, France, Germany, Spain, Holland, and Japan.

Result and Conclusion

Except for above mentioned seven copies, we found ten copies of the original edition as listed in Table 2. Therefore, seventeen original copies are extant in the world so far.

Acknowledgement

We would like to express our deep appreciation to the followings:
Dr. Vincent Collins, M.D., Department of Anesthesiology, University

Table 2 Ten Original Copies Discovered by Our Census

1. British Museum Library (London, U.K.)
2. Library of the University of Edinburgh (Edinburgh, U.K.)
3. Medical and Biological Library, University College London (London, U.K.)
4. Library of Royal College of Physicians (London, U.K.)
5. The Bryn Thomas Memorial Library (Reading, U.K.) [4]
6. Biblioteque Nationale (Paris, France)
7. Francis A Countway Library of Medicine (Boston, U.S.A.)
8. Moody Medical Library, University of Texas at Galveston (Galveston, U.S.A.)
9. Norman Library of Science and Medicine (San Francisco, U.S.A.)
10. Catalogue 21 of Medicine and the Life Sciences (Norman Company, U.S.A.) (presentation copy to Joshua Parsons)

of Illinois College of Medicine at Chicago, U.S.A., Francis A Countway Library of Medicine, Boston, U.S.A., Welcome Institute for the History of Medicine Library, London, U.K., Wood Libarary–Museum of Anesthesiology, Park Ridge, U.S.A., Woodward Biomedical Library, Vancouver, Canada.

References

1. Horowitz M and Collins J. A census of copies of the first edition of Andreas Vesalius' *De humani corporis fabrica* (1543), with a note on the recently discovered variant issue. J Hist Med All Sci 1984; 39: 189.
2. Keynes G. *Bibliography of the writings of Dr. William Harvey* (3rd ed.), revised by Whitteridge G and English C. Winchester, St. Paul's Bibliographies, 1989.
3. Ellis RH (ed.). *John Snow: On Narcotism by the Inhalation of Vapours*. London, Royal Society of Medicine Service, 1991.
4. The Bryn Thomas Collection of Historical Books on Anaesthesia –A catalogue –. Anaesthesia 1981;36:722.

2   The First Three Days in the History of Surgical Anesthesia in England

Matsuki A and Zsigmond EK
Anaesthesia 1973 ; 28 : 176–178.

It is generally accepted that the first successful administration of ether anaesthesia in England was in London on 19 December 1846 when, at the direction of Dr Boott, Dr J. Robinson anaesthetized a Miss Lonsdale, who was Dr Boott's niece, and a molar tooth was extracted. Two days later Professor Liston performed an amputation and avulsion of the great toes under ether at University College Hospital.

Dr Boott received information about a new method of mitigating pain during surgery from his friend, Professor Bigelow of Boston. The letter dated 28 November 1846 was brought to Liverpool by the Acadia, one of the four wooden paddle steamers belonging to the Cunard Company, which sailed from New York on 1 December and reached Liverpool on 16 December 1846.

Many authors[1–5] have made extensive searches in an attempt to ascertain when Dr Boott received the letter from Dr Bigelow and when it was that Dr Boott communicated the news of the discovery of anaesthesia to Dr Robinson but, until the present time, the answers to these questions have remained unknown. The authors were, therefore, extremely interested to find an important reference to this problem in an article written by Dr Robinson in 1855 in the *American Journal of Dental Science* (New Series).[6] The paper is entitled *Anaesthesia in Dental Surgery –Its history and introduction into Europe* and, so far as is known, no reference has been made to it in the various histories of anaesthesia. The following is an extract from the article:

> While these investigations were proceeding at the Massachusetts Hospital at Boston, my esteemed friend, Dr F. Booth [sic] received a private communication from Dr Bigelow, dated Boston, November 28th, 1846, in which he informed him of 'a new anodyne process lately introduced here, which promises to be one of the most important discoveries of the present age······ consisting of the inhalation of the vapor of ether to the point of intoxication, rendering the patient insensible to pain during surgical

operations, and other causes of suffering.'

The above extract from the private letter to Dr Booth [sic] with a newspaper report, constituted the whole of the intelligence on the effects of ether received in England on the 17th December, 1846. Dr Booth communicated this intelligence to myself and others on the 19th, at his house, and in the presence of his family, I etherized a young lady and extracted a molar tooth; this was the first operation, under the influence of ether, performed in England, which was subsequently reported to the medical journals; in a few days I introduced the agent at several of the metropolitan hospitals, and employed it for dental operations in my own practice.

Discussion

It would take 2 days for Dr Boott to prepare ether and an inhaler. Dr Robinson stated that the letter was 'received in England on December 17th.' This obviously means that Dr Boott received the letter on 17 December; it had actually arrived at Liverpool in the Acadia on the previous day.

Dr Boott having read Professor Bigelow's letter and the extract from the article written by Dr H. J Bigelow,[7] Professor Bigelow's son, in the Boston Medical and Surgical Journal, which described many hundreds of teeth extractions, thought he should select dental surgery for the first trial, chose Miss Lonsdale, who was suffering toothache, for the patient and asked Dr Robinson, a dentist, to administer ether and perform the operation on 19 December.

The introduction of ether to Scotland

It is very interesting that on the same day, 19 December, Dr William Scott used ether for surgical anaesthesia in Dumfries in Scotland.[8] He was informed of ether anaesthesia by his friend Dr William Fraser, who was the ship's surgeon of the Acadia. Dr Fraser hurried to his home town of Dumfries to report the news of the recent discovery to Dr Scott as soon as he arrived in port. Fraser reached Dumfries on 17 or 18 December and Dr Scott stated that he carried out surgery under ether anaesthesia within 48hr of receiving his report.[9] Dr Scott then wrote to Dr Buchanan of Glasgow and he and a dentist, also named Buchanan, carried out minor surgery under ether on Dr Buchanan's son on 22 or 23 December.

Summary

A recently discovered paper in the *American Journal of Dental Science* of 1855 throws new light on the chronology of the introduction of ether into England.

References

1. Keys, TE. (1945) *The History of Surgical Anesthesia*. Schuman, New York.
2. Duncum, B. M. (1947) *The Development of Inhalation Anaesthesia*, 1st ed. Oxford University Press, London.
3. Dawkins, C. J. (1947) The first public operation carried out under an anaesthetic in Europe. *Anaesthesia*, 2, 51.
4. Fulton, J. F. (1946) The reception in England of Henry Jacob Bigelow's original paper on surgical anesthesia. *New England Journal of Medicine*, 235, 745.
5. Sykes, W. S. (1960) The beginning of things. In: *Essays on the First Hundred Years of Anaesthesia*, 1st edn, Vol. 1, p. 48. Livingstone, Edinburgh.
6. Robinson, J. (1855) Anaesthesia in dental surgery–its history and introduction into Europe. *American Journal of Dental Science* (*New Series*), 5, 178.
7. Bigelow, H. J. (1846) Insensibility during surgical operations produced in inhalation. *Boston Medical and Surgical Journal*, 35, 309.
8. Baillie, T. W. (1965) The first European trial of anaesthetic ether. The Dumfries claim. *British Journal of Anaesthesia*, 37, 952.
9. Scott, W. (1872) The exhibition of ether as an anaesthetic. *Lancet*, ii, 585.

(Reproduced with the kind permission from the journal *Anaesthesia*.)

3   The First Published Report of Morton's Ether Anesthesia in the British Isles

Matsuki A and Zsigmond EK
Anaesthesist 1973 ; 22 : 389–392.

Summary. The history of surgical anesthesia has advanced into new era since William Morton demonstrated a successful ether anesthesia to a patient named Gilbert Abbot, who received surgery at the Massachusetts General Hospital on October 16, 1846. This epoch–making news spread rapidly across the Atlantic to European countries. According to Sykes and Davison, the first to report this information to Europe was Dr. Bigelow of Boston, and the first medical press mention of this was in The Lancet on December 26, 1846. However, the authors elucidated, by careful survey of numerous medical journals published in the year of 1846 and 1847, that the first bibliography describing Morton's ether anesthesia was the London Medical Gazette on December 18, 1846. One of the first to report this news to Europe was Dr. J.C. Warren, the very surgeon who performed the operation on Gilbert Abbot anesthetized by Morton on October 16, 1846.

The history of surgical anesthesia has advanced into a new era, since William Thomas Morton demonstrated a successful ether anesthesia to a patient named Gilbert Abbot operated on by John Collins Warren on October 16, 1846 at the Massachusetts General Hospital [1] [2], Davison [3] divided the history of anesthesia into seven epochs with the modern beginning in the year of 1846. The first performance by Morton is considered as a beacon–light not only for surgeons, who previously had no effective methods of eliminating pain and therefore, insufficient operative conditions, but also for millions of surgical patients who were previously operated on without "anesthesia."

This epoch–making news spread rapidly across the Atlantic to European countries. According to Beecher et al. [4] the news reached England less than six months after Morton's performance, but Davison [3] did not concur and stated H. J. Bigelow's letter, written on November 28, 1846, reached Dr. Boott in London in three weeks. The latter immediately sent a communication to the Lancet and wrote to Robert Liston, then Professor of Clinical Surgery in the University of London. W. S. Sykes [5], who studied in depth the first reference in Europe to Morton's ether anesthesia, stated, "All this, of course, was before the news of the great discovery had reached the Old World at all. The very first mention of anesthesia on the European side of the Atlantic was a tiny paragraph in the weekly supplement to the Liverpool Mercury, Friday, December 18th, 1846. A method of mitigating pain in surgical operations by the inhalation of certain ethers has been discovered in America, and it is said that successful experiments have been made."

Although studies by Sykes did not sufficiently elucidate this historical event, this report initiated out historical review.

Original [London Medical Gazette [6]
Animal Magnetism Superseded–Discovery of a New Hypnopoietic

We learn on the authority of a highly respectable physician of Boston, U. S., that a Dr. Morton, a surgeon–dentist of that city, has discovered a process whereby in a few minutes the most profound sleep may be induced, during which teeth may be extracted, and severe operations performed, without the patient being sensible of pain, or having any knowledge of the proceedings of the operator. The process simply consists in causing the patient to inhale the vapour of ether for a short period, and the effect is to produce complete insensibility, – or, as the writer says, intoxication. We quote the following case on the same respectable authority: "I took my daughter last week to Morton's rooms to have tooth extracted. She inhaled the (vapour of) ether about one minute and fell asleep instantly in the chair. A molar tooth was then extracted without the slightest movement of a muscle or fibre. In another minute the awoke, smiled, and said the tooth was not out, had felt no pain, nor the slightest knowledge of extraction. It was an entire illusion."

The facts are here so candidly stated that any one may put the new process to the test of experiment. Dr. Morton has made no mystery of his proceedings, like the tribe of hypnotic quacks who have lately perambulated the country. Some caution must, however, be observed in employing the vapour of ether in the way suggested. Ether is a strong narcotic, and its vapour speedily produces complete lethargy and coma: it is exceedingly volatile, and rapidly absorbed and diffused through the body, especially when brought into contact with the extensive surface of the air–cells of the lungs. In one case it has destroyed life, and in another caused apoplexy. Thus an individual may not awaken so readily as the young lady whose case we here quoted. It must be regarded as producing a state of temporary poisoning in which the nervous system is most powerfully affected; and as in concussion or narcotic poisoning, sensibility may be so destroyed that operations which in the healthy state would occasion severe pain, may be performed without any consciousness on the part of the patient. The respectability of the source from which we derive our information prevents us from doubting that the writer has accurately described what he saw. The awaking exactly one minute after the operation must of course be regarded as an accidental circumstance, depending on the dose of etheral vapour inhaled. One statement, however, appears to us to require explanation. We can understand the production of insensibility and the temporary loss of consciousness from the effects of ether; but we do not comprehend how, when the individual was perfectly roused to consciousness, there could be the slightest doubt as to whether the tooth was in or out of the mouth! All who have undergone this operation know that from the imperfect sense of touch possessed by the tongue, that the gap occasioned by the loss of a tooth appears about ten times as large as it really is. Then, again, we can believe that no pain might be felt during the operation; but how can any narcotic annihilate pain in future, when its effects on the nervous system have entirely ceased? Ordinary sleep often produces a temporary loss of sensation of pain; but this immediately returns in the waking state.

The date of this journal (December 18th, 1846) is the same as that of the supplement to the Liverpool Mercury. The former revealed the discoverer's name, method of the procedures and gave some comments on action and danger of the inhalation of ether. The latter mentioned only the fact that a method of mitigating pain during surgery was discovered in America.

There are two very important points to pay attention to. First, this report was communicated directly to the editor of The London Medical Gazette from someone in Boston who observed the actual demonstration by Morton, however, it is very regrettable that we lack the reporter's name and the date of communication. Secondly, the sentences, "I took my daughter last week ⋯⋯ It was an entire illusion" are quite the same as those of Dr. Bigelow's letter to Dr. Boott dated November 28th, 1846.

Considering these two points, the source is assumed to be Dr. Bigelow. There is little possibility that Dr. Boott sent this epoch–making news to The Lancet and The London Medical Gazette simultaneously. It is most probable that Dr. Bigelow reported this news to the editor of The London Medical Gazette and to Dr. Boott separately but almost simultaneously.

In any case, the above mentioned reference is the very first description of Morton's ether anesthesia to appear in the British Isles. This can be clearly confirmed by the following article [7] which appeared in The London Medical Gazette on January 1st, 1848.

The editor says:

> Since we gave the first public announcement in this country of the American discovery respecting the power of the vapour of ether to produce temporary narcotism, we have learned from an account given by Dr. Forbes that plan has been successfully tried by Mr. Liston at the University College Hospital.

This is followed by a description of Dr. Liston's operation and an extract from Dr. Bigelow's paper given by Dr. Forbes, which will be quoted below. At the end of this article, the editor notes as follows: "The reader will find an interesting summary of what is known concerning this singular discovery in the British and Foreign Medical Review for January, 1846." (You will see the year "1846" is an error and "1847" is correct.)

Dr. John Forbes, the editor of The British and Foreign Medical Review must have received some information concerning Morton's ether anesthesia, earlier than the editor of The Lancet who was informed by Dr. Boott. They included two personal communications directly addressed to him from his American friends in Boston and a copy of Dr. Bigelow's paper which appeared in The Boston Medical and Surgical Journal [8]. Dr. Forbes introduced this information under the title "On A New Means On Rendering Surgical Operations Painless" for the very last page of his journal published on January 1st, 1847 [9]. The authors quote the whole sentence, except for an extract from Dr. Bigelow's paper, since it is too important to neglect.

> On a New Means of Rendering Surgical Operations Painless
>
> Just as our last proof was passing through our hands, we received from our medical friends in Boston the account of a matter so interesting to surgeons, and indeed to everyone, that we take the opportunity of introducing it here. We know nothing more of this new method of eschewing pain that what is contained in the following extracts from two private letters, kindly written to us by our excellent friends, Dr. Ware and Dr. Warren, of Boston – both men of the highest eminence in their profession in America – and, we may truly say, in Europe also. It is impossible however, not to regard the discovery as one of the very highest

importance, not in the practice of operative surgery only, but also, as Dr. Ware suggests, in practical medicine also. We trust our friends will forgive us for putting into print their private communications. The importance of the subject and the necessity of authenticating the statements, are our excuses. The authors of the discovery are Dr. C. T. Jackson and Dr. Morton.

"Boston, November 29, 1846.

"I found, on my arrival here, a new thing in the medical world, or rather the new application of an old thing, of which I think you will like to hear. It is a mode of rendering patients insensible to the pain of surgical operations, by the inhalation of the vapour of the strongest sulphuric ether. They are thrown into a state nearly resembling that of complete intoxication from ardent spirits or of narcotism from opium. This state continues but a few minutes–five to ten–but, during it, the patient is insensible to pain. A thigh has been amputated, a breast extirpated, teeth drawn, without the slightest suffering. The number of operations of various kinds, especially those in dentistry, has been very considerable, and I believe but few persons resist the influence of the agent.

"The effect is not exactly the same on all. In some, the insensibility is entire, and the patient is aware of nothing which is going on ; in others, a certain degree of the power of perception remains, the patient knows what the operator is doing, perceives him for example, take hold of a tooth and draw it out, feels the grating of the instrument, but still has no pain.

"There are no subsequent ill effects to detract from the value of this practice, none even so great as those which follow a common dose of opium. One person told me she had some unpleasant sensations in the head for a short time, and was weak, languid, and faintish through the day, but not more so than she ordinarily was from having a tooth drawn. Another told me that he experienced something of the same kind and in addition that his breath smelt very strongly of ether for forty–eight hours, and was indeed so strongly impregnated with it as to affect the air of the room in which he sat, so as to be disagreeable to others.

"One of our best operative surgeons informs me that he regards it as chiefly applicable to cases of the large and painful operations which are performed rapidly, and do not require any very nice dissection, but that for the more delicate operations, which require some time, he would prefer to have the patient in his usual state. But it is impossible at present to judge what will be the limits to the application of such an agent. Objections may arise of which we do not dream, and evils may be found to follow, which we do not now perceive. Still it certainly promises much in surgery, and perhaps may be capable of application for other purposes beside the alleviation of pain. Would it not be worthy of trial in tetanus, in asthma, and in various cases of violent internal pain, especially from supposed spasms?

"It was brought into use by a dentist, and is now chiefly employed by that class of practitioners. He has taken out a patent for the discovery, and has despatched persons to Europe to secure one there also; so you will soon hear of it, and probably have an opportunity of witnessing its effects.

Faithfully yours, John Ware"

"Boston, November 24, 1846.
"You may have heard of the respiration of ether to prevent pain in surgical operations. In six cases I have had it applied with satisfactory success and no unpleasant sequel.
"I remain, & c, John C. Warren."

P. S. Dec. 22. –Yesterday we had ourselves the satisfaction of seeing this new mode of cheating pain put in practice by a master of chirurgery on our own side of the Atlantic. In the theatre of University College Hospital, Mr. Liston amputated the thigh of a man previously narcotised by inhalation of the ether vapour. Shortly after being placed on the operating table, the patient began to inhale, and became apparently insensible in the course of two or three minutes. The operation then commenced; and the limb was removed in what seemed to us a marvelously short space of time – certainly less than a minute; the patient remaining, during the incisions and the tying of the arteries, perfectly still and motionless. While the vessels were being secured, on being spoken to he roused partially up (still showing no signs of pain), and answered questions put to him in a slow, drowsy manner. He declared to us that at no part of the operation had he felt pain, though the seemed to be partially conscious; he heard some words, and felt that something was being done to his limb. He was not aware, till told, that the limb was off, and, when he knew it, expressed great gratification at having been saved from pain. The man seemed quite awake when removed from the operation–room, and continued so. Everything has since proceeded as usual, and very favorably. Mr. Liston afterwards performed one of the minor but most painful operations of surgery – the partial removal of the nail in onychia – on a man similarly narcotised, and with precisely the same result. The patient seemed to feel no pain, and, upon rousing up after the operation, declared that he had felt none.

In these cases the ether vapour was administered by means of an ingenious apparatus extemporaneously contrived by Mr. Squire, of Oxford Street. It consisted of the bottom part of a Nooth's apparatus, having a glass funnel filled with sponge soaked in pure washed ether, in the upper orifice, and one of Read's flexible inhaling tubes in the lower. As the ether fell through the neck of the funnel, it became vaporized, and the vapour being heavy, descended to the bottom of the vase, and was thence inspired through the flexible tube. No heat was applied to the apparatus or the ether.

The momentous details given above suggest many remarks which we have no room to record. We are only able to observe that if the new process shall supersede that employed, with a like object, by the mesmerists, we must concede to them that it supplies, from analogy, additional reasons for believing in their statements in regard to the production by their process, of insensibility to pain. (See Art. X, in our last Number). The readers of two articles in our last and present Numbers, will also observe the bearing of some of the present results on the semi-psychical discussions contained in them.

J. F.

Dr. J. C. Warren was the very surgeon of the Massachusetts General Hospital who performed an operation on Gilbert Abbot on "Ether Day." This article by Dr. Forbes seems very important in order to determine who was the first reporter of Morton's ether anesthesia to England. The date of the letter from Dr. Warren is November 24th, 1846, which is four days earlier than Dr. Bigelow's letter to Dr. Boott and five days earlier than Dr. Ware's letter to Dr. Forbes.

It remains unknown when and from whom the editor of The London Medical Gazette obtained the news. However, it can be said that one of the first reporters of this American discovery to England was Dr. J. C. Warren.
The title page of The Lancet dated December 26th, 1846, announced in advance the contents of The British and Foreign Medical Review, in which there was an article entitled, "On a New Means of Rendering Surgical Operations Painless." This would indicate to us that Dr. Forbes must have received the news earlier than the editor of The Lancet.

A brief paragraph of the last column of The Lancet dated December 26th, 1846 [10], quoted by Sykes as the first announcement in the medical press. It is not complete and is only half the original. The original is as shown below:

"Dr. Bigelow, of Boston, United States, has recently read a paper before one of the medical societies on a process for procuring insensibility to pain during surgical operations. Teeth in large numbers have been extracted, and even limbs amputated, without pain. Such a discovery, if it stands the test of examination, will be an invaluable boon. The means used is believed to be the inhalation of the vapour of sulphuric ether for two or three minutes, which, it is stated, produces insensibility for about an equal length of time. Dr. Bigelow is reported to have patented the process on the grounds that such an agent is capable of abuse – that its action is not thoroughly understood – and because it is looked forward to as of especial use in dentistry, many of whose process are secured by patient. Supposing the discovery to be genuine, even these offer but poor excuses for its reservation by patient."

This comment of the editor is full of criticism, while the editor of The London Medical Gazette gave a high evaluation. In addition to the above mentioned paragraph, there is one more paragraph on the same page, which Sykes neglected. It is as follows:

"Dr. Boott's important communication respecting Dr. Bigelow's discovery of a mode of producing insensibility during surgical operations, by the inhalation of sulphuric ether, shall be published next week."

References

1. Garrison, F. H.: An introduction to the history of medicine 4th ed. Philadelphia: Saunders 1929.
2. Keys, T. E.: The history of surgical anesthesia. New York: Schumans 1945.
3. Davison, M. H. A.: The evolution of anesthesia. Baltimore: Williams & Wilkins 1965.
4. Beecher, H., Ford, C.: Anesthesia. Fifty years progress, In: Fifty years of surgical progress, p. 225, ed. by L. Davis, The Franklyn Martin Memorial Foundation 1959.
5. Sykes, W. S.: Essays on the first hundred years of anesthesia, vol. I. Edinburgh: E. S. Livingstone 1960.
6. London Medical Gazette, (New Series) 3, 1085–1086 (1846). (December 18, 1846). J. F. Fulton stated this was the first reference in the British press to the use of ether in his paper entitled "The reception in England of Henry Jacob Bigelows original paper on surgical anesthesia." New Engl. J. Med. 235, 745–746 (1966).

7. London Medical Gazette. (New Series) 4, 38–39 (1847). (January 1, 1847).
8. Bigelow, H. J.: Insensibility during surgical operations produced by inhalation. Boston med. surg. J. 85, 309–317 (1846).
9. British and foreign med. Rev. 23, 309–312 (1847).
10. Lancet 1846 II, 704.

(Reproduced with kind permission from Springer.)

4   The Introduction of Chloroform Anesthesia in the United States

Matsuki A and Zsigmond EK
Anesth and Analg 1974 ; 54 : 148–152.

5   The First Fatal Case of Chloroform Anesthesia in the United States.

Matsuki A and Zsigmond EK
Anesth and Analg 1974 ; 53 : 152–154.

I was unable to obtain permissions from the publisher to reproduce above two articles due to some communication and computer troubles by the deadline for printing.

6   The First Fatal Case of Chloroform Anesthesia in Canada

Matsuki A and Zsigmond EK
Can Anaesth Soc J 1973 ; 20 : 395–397.

On January 28, 1848, only three months after James Young Simpson introduced chloroform in clinical anaesthesia,[1] the first fatal case due to the inhalation of chloroform occurred in the British Isles.[2] Thereafter, a number of deaths caused by chloroform inhalation occurred in succession. Lyman[3] stated that between 1848 and 1881, 393 fatal cases occurred during and following the inhalation of chloroform.

This anaesthetic was introduced to Canada in January 1848,[4,5] but ten years elapsed before the first fatality caused by administration of chloroform was reported.

Mr. John McChesney of Toronto went to Dr. French's office to have his teeth extracted on February 1, 1858. The patient was informed about chloroform anaesthesia and he agreed to inhale the agent at his own risk. Then Dr. Richardson, Dr. French's associate, administered the agent by applying a moistened sponge over the nostrils. When the doctor finished extracting six teeth, with some difficulty in the last tooth, the patient was still responsive to vocal orders. Death occurred instantaneously thereafter.

The details are reported in the column of the editorial department of the Medical Chronicle or Montreal Monthly Journal of Medicine and Surgery.[6] It reads as follows:

Death from Chloroform

   A painful feeling was lately occasioned in Toronto by the melancholy death of Mr. John McChesney. This gentleman called at the operating room of Dr. French, surgeon dentist, to have six teeth extracted, but appeared reluctant to submit to the operation unless under the influence of chloroform. Dr. Richardson was accordingly sent for to administer it, which he did, first, however, explaining to Mr. McChesney that he took the anaesthetic solely at his own risk. After a short inhalation, the gums were lanced, and the chloroform having been again applied, the teeth were removed. But as soon as this was done Mr. McChesney was seen to alter in appearance; his eyes became fixed, the jaws fell, respiration ceased, and the heart action stopped. Every possible attempt was made to restore animation but to no purpose: Mr. McChesney was dead. Fuller details respecting his death will be found in the evidence below, taken at the inquest held the same evening 1st February.

Dr. Tobias French, in reply to the foreman of the jury, described the manner in which Dr. Richardson administered the chloroform, by placing it in a sponge and applying it to the nostrils of the patient. After a short time, the patient began to laugh; asked him the cause, and he said he could not help it, seeing those fellows (meaning us) laughing at him. It was then thought he was sufficiently insensible to commence the operation of lancing the gums. He winced under the lancing; I asked him to lean forward and spit into the bowl, which he did. He did not speak, but groaned several times. I remarked to the Doctor, that he was getting on well. After a few inhalations, the Doctor said it was better to draw the teeth, and my brother did so. He extracted six. The deceased seemed conscious of pain, and struggled in the drawing of the last tooth, and appeared like a person not fully under the influence. I asked him to lean over the bowl, which I held before him, and he spat into it. I then observed a change pass over his countenance, such as to startle me; and I remarked there was something wrong. Dr. Richardson opened the window, and ordered me to tip the patient on the right side, so that he would not swallow any blood. I next remarked a great change, and exclaimed that he was gone. The deceased at this time looked cadaverous, and his jaw fell. We then took him and laid him on the floor, placed a pillow under his head, and made an application of ammonia; also applied cold water to his head, and had the body briskly rubbed. Dr. Richardson called for assistance and Drs. Russell, Nicholl, Beaumont, and Haswell were brought in. A galvanic battery was also put in operation; but all was of no avail.

Dr. Richardson was examined, and deposed that every precaution was taken in the case of Mr. McChesney, and quoted instances of a similar nature which had taken place in England.

Dr. Haswell. –When I went to Dr. French's I found the deceased lying on the floor. Respiration had then ceased. Dr. Richardson was using efforts to restore animation. I assisted, in conjunction with Drs. Beaumont and Nicholl, for about an hour.

At this stage of the proceedings, it was intimated by the jury that abundant medical testimony had been adduced, and no further evidence was taken.

After a short deliberation, the jury found the following verdict: "That the deceased came to his death in Dr. French's operating room, while under the influence of chloroform, which he had voluntarily inhaled for the purpose of getting some teeth extracted; and that more than ordinary care was used in the administration of the chloroform."

The patient was considered to have no problem immediately before the start of anaesthesia, as Dr. Richardson testified every precaution had been taken in this case. Anaesthesia was not so deep as to lose consciousness completely, and the patient could respond slightly to the doctor's verbal command. Considering these facts, it is most likely that the patient died of sudden cardiac arrest caused by influence of chloroform and not by asphyxia.

As far as the authors know, more than ten chloroform deaths were reported for a period from 1861 to 1897 in Canada.[7-17] In his paper in 1873, Dr. Coleman[18] of the Toronto Eye and Ear Infirmary discussed mode of death, cause of death, per cent of fatal cases, condition of patient, sign of danger, methods of administration and rules for administration in relation to chloroform anaesthesia.

According to the Editorial in the Canada Lancet, 1887,[19] the following factors were reported to be the important causes of so-called chloroform death: (i) paralysis of the respiratory center from an overdose; (ii) paralysis of the heart from a too concentrated chloroform vapor; and (iii) a combination of chloroform narcosis and shock.

The editors of the Canada Medical and Surgical Journal[20] attributed employment of chloroform instead of ether and incorrect resuscitation to the causes of so-called chloroform death. Chloroform was, however, still a popular inhalational anaesthetic at that time.

References

1. Simpson J. Y. On a new anesthetic agent, more efficient than sulphuric ether. Lancet, 2: 349–550 (1847).
2. Fatal Application of Chloroform. Lancet 1: 161–162 (1848).
3. Lyman, H. M. Artificial anaesthesia and anaesthetics. New York. William Wood and Company, 1881, pp.136–201.
4. Holmes, A. F. Employment of chloroform. Brit. Amer. J. Med. Phys. Sci. 3: 263–264 (1848).
5. Worthington, E. D. Cases of chloroform. Brit. Amer. J. Med. Phys. Sci. 3: 326–327 (1848).
6. The Medical Chronicle or Montreal Monthly Journal of Medical and Surgery. 5: 425–427 (1858).

7. Roland, C. G. The first death from chloroform at the Toronto General Hospital. Can. Anaes. Soc. J., 11: 437–439 (1964).
8. Canad. Med. J. (Montreal) 3: 380 (1867).
9. Death from chloroform. Canad. Med. Record. 6: 20 (1877–78).
10. Death from chloroform. Canad. Lancet 10: 157 (1878).
11. Death from chloroform. Canad. Lancet 11: 313 (1879).
12. Death from chloroform. Canad. Lancet 12: 157–158 (1880).
13. Another death from chloroform. Canad. Lancet 12: 349 (1880).
14. Caviller, A. C. The case of sudden death during the first stage of chloroform inhalation. Canad. Lancet 13: 231–232 (1881).
15. LaCross, E. Death under chloroform. Montreal Medical J. 19: 919–920 (1881).
16. Death from chloroform. Canad. Lancet 25: 127 (1883).
17. Death from chloroform. Canad. Practioner 18: 309 (1893).
18. Coleman, W. S. The administration of chloroform. Canad. Lancet 5: 616–624 (1872–3).
19. Death from chloroform. Canad. Lancet 29: 281–282 (1887).
20. Chloroform deaths. Canad. Medical Surgical J. 16: 248–249 (1887).

(Reproduced with kind permission from Springer.)

7 A Chronology of the Very Early History of Inhalation Anesthesia in Canada

Matsuki A
Canad Anaesth Soc J 1974 ; 21 : 92–95.

Although several well documented articles[1-7] are available on the history of surgical anaesthesia in Canada, it has not been fully elucidated when information about ether anaesthesia was first brought from the United States to Canada. Furthermore, the available sources contain conflicting reports as to who administered the first surgical anaesthetic with ether and chloroform, as well as the first obstetrical anaesthetic.

Fuller[2] states that Dr. Almon was the first to use chloroform for surgical anaesthesia; yet Shields[5] attributes the first chloroform anaesthetic to Dr. A. F. Holmes. According to a recent article by Jacques,[6] Dr. Worthington was the first to administer both ether and chloroform during surgical operations. McKenzie[1] and Fuller[2] report that a chemist, Frazer, of Nova Scotia, administered chloroform to his wife during delivery and that consequently this was the first obstetrical anaesthetic. However, Heagerty[3] credits Dr. Holmes with its first use for parturition in Canada. Thus it is still unclear exactly when, where and who administered the first surgical and obstetrical anaesthetics with ether or chloroform in Canada.

It seems appropriate, therefore, to provide a chronology of the history of early surgical anaesthesia in Canada, in the hope that this may be helpful to future historians.

November, 1846.
Information on ether anaesthesia is brought to Canada.
The British American Journal of Medicine and Physical Science (Brit. Amer. J. 2: 226, 1846 Dec. 1, 1846) announces in the column of "Books etc. Received during the Month" that they have received the November issue of the Boston Medical and Surgical Journal which includes H. J. Bigelow's paper on ether anaesthesia.

January, 1847.
First mention of ether anaesthesia appears in Canadian Medical Journal.
First mention of ether anaesthesia entitled "Insensibility During Surgical

Operations Produced by Inhalation" appears in a Canadian Journal. This is an extract from the December (1846) issue of the Philadelphia Medical Examiner. (Brit. Amer. J. 2: 247 (1847).)

January, 1847.
Dr. Nelson begins experiments with ether anaesthesia.
Mr. Webster, a dentist of Montreal, purchases an ether inhaler from a "chevalier d'industrie." Mr. Webster and Dr. Horace Nelson begin experiments with ether anaesthesia using dogs and also administer it to each other. (Brit. Amer. J, 3: 34 (1847).)

March, 1847.
Dr. J. Douglass employs ether for the amputation of toes (the first use of ether anaesthesia in Canada).
Dr. James Douglass of Quebec amputates the toes of a man under ether anaesthesia. This anaesthetic precedes the one to Dr. Nelson's patient. (Brit. Amer. J. 2: 338 (1847).)

March, 1847.
Mr. Webster successfully administers ether to Dr. Nelson's patient.
Dr. Wolfred Nelson (Horace Nelson's father) succeeds in removing a large tumour from a woman. Mr. Webster anaesthetizes her with ether. The date of the operation is unknown, but took place before March 8, 1847. (Brit. Amer. J. 3: 34 (1847).)

March 11, 1847.
Dr. Worthington employs ether anaesthesia.
Dr. Worthington of Sherbrooke amputates the foot of a 30–year–old man using ether anaesthesia. He employs a large ox–bladder with a stop–cock as an inhaler. (Brit. Amer. J. 3: 10 (1847).)

March, 1847.
Dr. Campbell's failure with ether anaesthesia.
Dr. Campbell fails to anaesthetize a patient with ether at the Montreal General Hospital. (Brit. Amer. J. 2: 338 (1847).)

March, 1847.
Editorial on anaesthesia appears in Brit. Amer. J.
The editorial "Inhalation of Sulphuric Ether Vapour" appears in the March

issue of the British American Journal. (Brit. Amer. J. 2: 304 (1847).)

September 6, 1847.
Dr. Crawford uses ether for tetanus.
Dr. J. Crawford of McGill College uses ether for sedating a patient with traumatic tetanus. (Brit. Amer. J. 3: 199 (1847).)

November, 1847.
Dr. J. Crawford administers successful ether anaesthesia.
Dr. J. Crawford uses ether anaesthesia successfully for the amputation of the leg of a 14–year–old boy at the Montreal General Hospital. (Brit. Amer. J. 3: 199 (1847).)

January 24, 1848.
Dr. Worthington uses chloroform (the first use of chloroform anaesthesia in Canada).
Dr. E. D. Worthington of Sherbrooke employs chloroform to alleviate pain during the manual reduction of a fracture of the femur in an old woman. The pain relief is only partial. (Brit. Amer. J. 3: 326 (1848).)

January 25, 1848.
Dr. E. D. Worthington succeeds in removing a tumour from the right hand of a child under chloroform anaesthesia. (Brit. Amer. J. 3: 326 (1848).)

January 25, 1848.
Dr. Holmes gives successful obstetrical anaesthesia with chloroform (the first use of chloroform for childbirth in Canada).
Dr. A. F. Holmes, Professor of the Theory and Practice of Medicine, McGill College, Montreal, uses chloroform anaesthesia successfully in a case of parturition. (Brit. Amer. J. 3: 263 (1848).)

January, 1848.
Dr. Sutherland administers chloroform anaesthesia in Montreal.
Dr. Sutherland of the Montreal General Hospital performs anaesthesia successfully. The operation took place between January 23 and January 29. (Brit. Amer. J. 3: 278 (1848).)

February 1, 1848.
Dr. Almon administers chloroform anaesthesia.

Dr. W. J. Almon of Halifax amputates the thumb of a woman under chloroform anaesthesia in the presence of Dr. Parker and Dr. Brown. (Canad. Med. Assoc. J. 14: 254 (1924).)

February 3, 1848.
Dr. Martin reports three cases of chloroform anaesthesia. Dr. J. Martin of the Quebec Marine Hospital performs three operations under chloroform anaesthesia. The first two are amputations of the great toes of Francis McNamara, aged 18 and Denis O'Hara aged 16. The third is an amputation of both legs of Adam Belte, a French sailor. (Brit. Amer. J. 3: 325 (1848).)

February 4, 1848.
Dr. Marsden mentions two cases of chloroform anaesthesia.
Dr. W. Marsden of Quebec reports two cases of chloroform anaesthesia. The first case is an amputation of both legs of Pierre Francois Lamane, aged 33, by Dr. J. Douglass and Dr. A. Sewell. The second case is a tonsillectomy performed on a 14–year–old boy by Dr. J. Douglass. (Brit. Amer. J. 3: 288 (1848).)

February 12, 1848.
Dr. Nelson undertakes lithotomy during chloroform anaesthesia.
Dr. W. Nelson of Montreal performs a lithotomy on a man aged 65 under chloroform anaesthesia. Dr. Arnoldi and Dr. Sutherland assist at the operation. (Lancet, 1: 380 (1848).)

February 15, 1848.
Dr. Johnstone uses chloroform for delivery.
Dr. James B. Johnstone of Sherbrooke reports three cases of chloroform anaesthesia during parturition. (Brit. Amer. J. 3: 324 (1848).)

March 10, 1848.
Dr. Almon's chloroform anaesthesia.
Dr. W. J. Almon of Halifax amputates the leg of a woman under chloroform anaesthesia. (Canad. Med. Assoc. J. 14: 254 (1924).)

March 22, 1848.
Dr. Frazer administers chloroform to his wife.
A chemist, D.B. Frazer of Pictou, Nova Scotia, administers chloroform to his wife during delivery. Chloroform used is manufactured by himself.

(Canad. Pharmaceutical J. 58: 118 (1924).)

May 31, 1848.
Dr. Campbell's chloroform anaesthesia.
Dr. Duncan Campbell removes a breast tumour under chloroform anaesthesia. (Canad. Med. Assoc. J. 32: 84 (1935).)

February 1, 1858.
First anaesthetic death in Canada.
Mr. John McChesney dies suddenly following chloroform anaesthesia in the operating room of Dr. French of Montreal. This is the first death under chloroform anaesthesia. (Medical Chronicle 5: 425 (1858).)

References

1. Mackenzie, K. A. Early adventures with chloroform in Nova Scotia. C. M. A. J. 1928, 14: 254–255 (1924).
2. Fuller, R. C. & Amhehst, N. S. The first anaesthetic record of the use of chloroform on this side of the Atlantic. Canad. Pharaceu. J. 58: 118–119 (1924).
3. Heagerty, J. J. Four centuries of medical history in Canada. Macmillan 1928. Vol. 1, pp. 304–307.
4. Colebeck, W. K. The first record of an anaesthetic in Ontario. C. M. A. J. 32: 84–85 (1935).
5. Shields, H. J. The history of anaesthesia in Canada. Canad. Anaes. Soc. J. 2: 301–307 (1955).
6. Jacques, A. The Hotel Dieu de Quebec. 1634–1964. Anaesth. Analg. 45: 15–20 (1966).
7. Ibid: anaesthesia in Canada 1847–1967. The beginning of anaesthesia in Canada. Canad. Anaes. Soc. J. 14: 500–509 (1967).

(Reproduced with kind permission from Springer.)

8   A Bibliography of the History of Surgical Anaesthesia in Canada
   – Supplement to Dr. Roland's checklist –

Matsuki A and Zsigmond EK
Canad Anaesth Soc J 1974 ; 21 : 427–430.

Canada was one of the earliest countries to introduce ether anaesthesia. Canadian physicians have contributed much to progress in the field. However, the history of surgical anaesthesia in Canada has not been fully documented.

The present bibliography is a supplement to Roland's preliminary checklist, which lacks many important articles published before 1900.[1] Hopefully it will augment studies of the history of surgical anaesthesia in Canada.

GENERAL

Editorial Note: Books etc. received during the month. Brit. Amer. J. Med. Phys. 2: 226 (1846).
   This shows Boston Medical and Surgical J. including Bigelow's paper on ether anaesthesia is brought to Canada as early as in November 1846.

Medical News: Employment of Chloroform in Canada. Lancet (London) 1: 350 (1848).
   Report on Dr Nelson's lithotomy on a man under the influence of chloroform anaesthesia on February 12, 1848.

Editorials: The Jubilee of Anaesthesia. Canad. Practitioner 21 : 844–845 (1896).

Fuller, R. C. & Amherst, N. S. The first authentic record of the use of chloroform on this side of the Atlantic. Canad. Pharmaceut. J. 58: 118–119 (1924).
   The content is almost the same as MacKenzie's article. Dr Almon was not the first to use chloroform, Dr C. Harris of Baltimore used it for the first time outside the British Isles on about Dec. 19, 1847.

Muir, W. L. President's Address, Canadian Society of Anaesthetists. Canadian Practitioner 49: 420–426 (1924).

> In this article, Muir describes how Dr Ingaris performed an operation under anaesthesia produced by laudanum and rum. Muir also describes chloroform anaesthesia by Dr Almon and Mr Frazer.

Johnston, S. The growth of the specialty of anaesthesia in Canada. Canad. Med. A. J. 17: 163–165 (1927).

Webster, W. Notes on the development of anaesthesia in Western Canada. Canad. Med. Assoc. J. 17: 727–728 (1927).
> Brief comment on the history of anaesthesia in Winnipeg and Vancouver.

Rolland, P. L'evolution de l'anesthesie. J. Canad. Dent. A. 8: 47–54 (1946).
> General history of anaesthesia.

Shields, H. J. Account of the history of anaesthesia in Canada. Brit. M. J. 2: 129 (1955).

Ghiffith, H.R. Fifty years of progress in surgery and anaesthesia. Canad. Nurse 54: 540–542 (1958).

ANAESTHETICS

Editorial Note: Chloroform. Brit. Amer. J. Med. Phys. Sci. 3: 278 (1848).
> "Two instances of the application of this anaesthetic agent have occurred in this city within the last week – one a case of parturition, reported in this number by Dr Holmes, the other an amputation at the Montreal General Hospital, by which its soporific powers were most successfully brought into play. This case, we hope, will be reported also, and we therefore forbear anticipating any of Dr Sutherland's remarks on it. From what we have seen, we consider it as more valuable in its effects than ether, and (which is of some moment) less expensive. It is easily prepared; and for the benefit of our country subscribers, who may have difficulty in obtaining it from this city, in which it is largely manufactured by S. J. Lyman and Co., we give the following formula: Take of chloride of Lime four ounces, Alcohol one ounce, Water twelve ounces–mix in a capacious retort/ and distil with a moderate heat. Two fluids come over, one of which, oily and heavier than the other, collects at the bottom of the receiver properly adapted to the retort. This is the Chloroform, and requires to be separated by in the first instance, a decantation of the super-natant fluid, and to be purified and rectified, in the second, by a re-distillation from Chloride of Calcium. The quantity thus obtained is small. The secret of its economical manufacture consists in the employment of large quantities of the materials. We refer our readers

to the Periscopic Department for fuller quotations from our British exchanges on the subjects."

Campbell, F. W. On the Administration of Chloroform. Canad. Med. J 1: 157–161 (1865).

Rosebrugh, A. M. Chloroform. Dominion M. J. 1: 64 (1868–9), 2: 84 (1869–70).

Atherton, A. B. On the exhibition of chloroform. Canad. Lancet 5: 114–116 (1872–3).

Editorial: Ether Chloroform. Canad. Lancet 5: 256–258 (1872–3).

Carey, R. H. On the advantages of ether over chloroform as an anaesthetic agent. Canad. Lancet 5: 331–334 (1872–3).

Coleman, W. S. The administration of chloroform. Canad. Lancet 5: 616–624 (1872–3).

    Nice review article on chloroform anaesthesia.

Pope, J. W. Chloroform in heart disease. Canad. Med. Rec. 2: 189 (1873–74).

Saint–Germain, M. De. Anaesthesia in children. Canad. J. Med. Sci. 4: 48–54 (1879).

Hingston, W. H. Certain anaesthetics. Canad. Med. Rec. 8: 225–228 (1880).

Editorial: Ether as an Anaesthetic. Canad. Lancet 10: 62 (1878).

MacDonnell, R. L. The administration of chloroform. Canad. Med. Surg. J. 9: 11–19 (1880–81).

    This paper mentions almost fatal cases of chloroform anaesthesia.

Gaynoh, J. J. Chloroform as an anaesthetic – Its physiological action and therapeutic value. Canad. Lancet 16: 65–70 (1883).

    This article describes physiological action and mentions 13 substantial rules when giving chloroform anaesthesia.

Wood. C. A. Notes on the use of ether in obstetrics. Canad. Med. Rec. 12: 73–76 (1884).

    A total of 26 cases of obstetrical anaesthesia are mentioned.

Editorial: Our Choice of Anaesthetics. Canad. Practitioner 10: 150–151 (1885).

    This gives eight general rules for administration of anaesthetics.

Smith, L. The A.C.E. mixture. The best anaesthetic in obstetrical practise. Canad. Med. Rec. 14: 337–341 (1885).

    A mixture which is composed of alcohol, chloroform and ether, in proportions of 1, 2 and 3 of each, respectively, is highly recommended for obstetrical anaesthesia.

Editorial: Local Anaesthetics. Mont. Med. J. 17: 226–227 (1888).

Editorial: Anaesthesia by Chloroform. Canad. Practioner 17: 334 (1892).

Balfour, J. D. Administration of chloroform and the dangers incident hitherto. Montreal Med. J. 21 : 663–676 (1892–93).

Campbell, G. G. The pulse and respiration during ether anaesthesia with Clover's inhaler. Canad. Med. Rec. 23: 71–81 (1894–5).

Campbell, G. G. Anaesthesia in a case with diminished breathing area. Mont. Med. J. 24: 18–19 (1895–6).

Freeman, J. Chloroform or Ether? Canad. Practitioner 21 : 581–587 (1896).

Scadding, H. C. The selection of an anaesthetic. Canad. Practitioner 23: 84–87 (1898).

G. S. R.: A suggestion for anaesthetics. Canad. Practitioner 24: 357 (1899).
"I have been in the habit for the past two years of having a little eau de cologne or other perfume dropped on the inhaler to begin with; then a few minutes chloroform is added."

COMPLICATIONS

Editorial: Death from chloroform. Medical Chronicle (Montreal) 5: 425–427 (1858).
This first death due to chloroform anaesthesia occurred on February 1, 1858. Editorial: Death from chloroform. Canad. M. J. 3: 380 (1867).

Saundehs, H. J. Remarks on a case of chloroform poisoning. Canad. Lancet 6: 209–210 (1873–74).

Wade, W. Nelaton's method of resuscitation from chloroform narcosis – successful case. Canad. Lancet 7: 165–166 (1875).

Coverton, C.W. Successful case of resuscitation from chloroform narcotics. Nelaton's Method. Canad. Lancet 7: 193–194 (1875).

News: Death from chloroform. Canad. Med. Rec. 6: 20 (1877).
Death occurred by chloroform anaesthesia in Toronto General Hospital on July 18, 1877.

News: Death from chloroform. Canad. Lancet 10: 157 (1878).

News: Death from chloroform. Canad. Lancet 11: 313 (1879).

Editorials: Death from chloroform. Canad. Lancet 12: 157–158 (1880).

News: Another death from chloroform. Canad. Lancet 12: 349 (1880).

Woolverton, A. Death under ether. Canad. Med. Surg. J. 9: 508–509 (1880–1).

LaCrosse, E. Death under chloroform. Montreal Med. J. 19: 919–920 (1880–81).

Gartller, A. C. The case of sudden death during the first stage of chloroform. Canad. Lancet13: 231–232 (1881).

Atherton, A. B. Case of chloroform poisoning. Canad. Lancet 13: 301–302

(1881).

Nelson, C. E. Dangerous inhalation of nitrous oxide gas. Canad. Med. Rec. 9: 193–194 (1881).

News: Death from chloroform. Canad. Lancet 15: 127 (1883).

Editorial: Chloroform death. Canad. Med. Surg. J. 16: 248–249 (1887).

"Two grave mistakes were made: 1st, the employment of chloroform instead of ether. 2nd, the failure to use those means which science has demonstrated to be the most efficacious in restoring a failing Circulation."

Editorial: Death from chloroform. Canad. Lancet 19: 281–282 (1887).

"The danger of anaesthetics are chiefly three, viz: paralysis of the respiratory centre, from an overdose, paralysis of the heart, from a too concentrated chloroform vapor and a combination of chloroform narcosis and shock."

Editorials: Death from chloroform. Canad. Practitioner 28: 309 (1893).

Ross, J. F. W. Heart from chloroform poisoning case. Canad. Practitioner 21: 437–438 (1896).

Editorials: Danger of chloroform. Canad. Practitioner 22: 382–383 (1897).

William, J. A. Inertia of the uterus following the use of chloroform. Canad. Practitioner 22: 436 (1897).

Editorials : Death from chloroform. Canad. Practitioner 22: 209–210 (1897).

Rudolf, R. D. A note on death from chloroform. Canad. Practitioner 23: 82–83 (1898).

Oldright, H. H. Anaesthesia and analgesia. Dominion Medical Monthly 10: 134–136 (1898).

MISCELLANEOUS

O'Reilly, C. Anaesthetic requirements. Canad. J. Med. Surg. 1: 154 (1897).
Possibly the first anaesthesia chart in Canada. A revised anaesthesia chart appeared in 1901. Canad. Lancet 34: 636–637 (1901).

Cassedy, J. J. Anaesthetic requirements. Canad. J. Med. Surg. 1: 176 (1897).
Brief comment on O'Reilly's anesthesia chart.

Editorial: The compensation of the anaesthetist. Dominion Med. Monthly 14: 87–88 (1900).

"Where an operator receives $20.00 for an operation, his assistant the joyful recipient of probably $20.00 to $25.00, and the poor anaesthetist $5.00 with perhaps in some cases $10.00."

Abrahams, S. On oxygen gas as an antidote to the deleterious effects of anaesthetic agents. Canad. Med. J. 1: 667 (1852–53).

Reference

1. Roland, C. G. Bibliography of The History of Anaesthesia in Canada: Preliminary checklist. Canad. Anaesth. Soc. J. 15: 202 (1968).

(Reproduced with kind permission from Springer.)

9 The Early Anesthesia Chart in Canada

Matsuki A and Zsigmond EK
Anaesthesist 1974 ; 23 : 268–269.

Although several articles [1–3] are available concerning the history of surgical anesthesia in Canada, it is still unknown to us when an anesthesia chart was first used in this country. Roland [4] described that an anesthesia chart arranged by Dr. O'Reilly had been used at the Toronto General Hospital in 1901.

The author found and has reproduced below (Table 1) Dr. O'Reilly's original chart which bears the early date 1897 [5].

The following three anesthetic requirements were added to the revised chart which appeared in 1901; feathers for tube, nitro–glycerine 1/100 gr and saline solution; 3i to 0i. J. C. Cassidy [6], editor of the Canadian Journal of Medicine and Surgery recommended the use of the chart to future medical writers.

Table 1. Toronto General Hospital

Anaesthetic Requirements		
Instruments	Restoratives	Miscellaneous
Tongue Forceps	Liq. Anm. Fort.	Wax Candle and Matches
Mouth Gag	Spts. Amm. Arom't.	Towels for Friction
Tongue Depressor	Brandy and Whiskey	Large Fan
Sponge and Holder	Liq. Strychniae	Hot Water Bottles, Cold Water
Tracheotomy Tube	Ether	Blocks or Bricks to elevate foot of Table
Tracheotomy Knife	Tr. Digitalis	Ice, for rectum
Hypodermic Syringes	Sol. Green Tea	Conical Jaw Opener
Oesophageal Forceps	Amyl. Nitrite Pearls	Forced Expiration Apparatus
Davidson Syringe	Oxygen Gas	Battery

Form to be Filled in Before the Administration of an Anaesthetic

Name .... Disease ....
Age .... Sex .... Birthplace ....
Occupation .... Ward No .... House Surgeon ....
Date of Admission .... Date of Discharge ....
Under care of .... Report taken by ....
Habits? Alcohol .... Diseases? Epilepsy ....
  Opium ....   Apoplexy ....
  Cocaine ....   Bright's Disease ....
  Other Drugs ....   Other Diseases ....

Patient's Condition

Pulse before............................ during........................... after....................
Circulation .... Heart ....
Lungs ....
Nervous System ....
Urinary Analysis – Sp. Gr. .... Albumin ....
        Reaction .... Sugar ....
Anaesthetic commenced at .... Discontinued at ....
Anaesthetic used .... Amount used ....
State of Stomach during operation ....
Return to consciousness at ....
Date .... Administrator .... M.D.

General Remarks

Noticeable and still unfamiliar to the modern anesthesiologists is the section entitled "Circulation". No section entitled "Blood Pressure" is included.

The reasons may be as follows: First, routine measurements of the arterial blood pressure was not easily done until Riva–Rocci [7] invented a new sphygmomanometer in 1896. Second, most surgeons considered it unnecessary to measure the arterial blood pressure during surgery [8]. Third, it was not until 1903 when Cushing and his associate [9] reported their influential paper concerning routine measurements in the operating room.

References

1. Heaguty, J. J.: Four Centuries of Medical History of Canada. Vol. 1. p.304 Toronto: MacMilan (1928)
2. Shields, H. J.: The History of Anaesthesia in Canada. Canad. Anaesth. Soc. J. 2, 301 (1955)
3. Jacques, A.: Anaesthesia in Canada, 1847–1967. 1. The Beginnings of Anaesthesia in Canada. Canad. Anaesth. Soc. J. 14, 500(1967)
4. Roland, C. G.: Bibliography of the History of Anesthesia in Canada: Preliminary Checklist. Canad. Anaesth. Soc. J. 15, 202–214(1968)
5. O'Reilly, C.: Anaesthetic Requirements. Canad. J. med. Surg. 1, 154 (1897)
6. Cassidy, J. C.: Anaesthetic Requirements. Canad. J. med. Surg. 1, 176 (1897)
7. Riva–Rocci, S.: A New Sphygmomanometer. from "Foundations of Anesthesia" by Faulconer, Jr. A. and Keys, T. E. Springfield: C. C. Thomas, 2, p.1053–1075 (1965)
8. Beecher, H. K.: The First Anesthesia Records (Codman, Cushing) Surg. Gynec. Obstet. 71, 689 (1940)
9. Cushing, H., Baltimore, M.: On Routine Determinations of Arterial Tension in Operating Room and Clinic. Boston Med. Surg. J. 148, 250–256 (1903)

(Reproduced with kind permission from Springer.)

10   The First Fatal Case of Chloroform Anaeshtesia in Australia

Matsuki A
Anaesthesia and Intensive Care 1973 ; 1 : 301–302.

It was only three months after Sir James Young Simpson introduced chloroform in clinical anaesthesia that the first fatal case due to chloroform anaesthesia occurred on 28th January, 1848 (Editorial 1848).

Thirteen deaths caused by chloroform inhalation were reported during a period of five years (1852–1856) and 57 deaths were reported during the six-year period 1863–1868 (Murray 1873). Lyman (1881) stated that between 1848 and 1881, 393 fatal cases occurred during or after the inhalation of chloroform.

The following is a newspaper report of what is considered to be the first death due to chloroform anaesthesia to occur in Australia. The news was brought to the editor of the Medical Times and Gazette (London), and it appeared in the column of Medical News of the journal of 20th November, 1852. It reads as follows:

Death From Chloroform in Australia

(From a Correspondent.) – An inquest was held yesterday at the Clarendon Hotel, Melbourne, before W. B. Wilmot, Esq., city coroner, on the body of Mr. John Atkinson, who was alleged to have died from the effects of chloroform. Mr. Morton, landlord of the Clarendon Hotel, stated that the deceased had been in the habit of staying at his house at intervals for the last three years. On the present occasion, he had been there about three weeks. Deceased told witness, three days previous to his death, that he was about to be operated on for fistula. The prospect of the operation did not appear to depress him, and he treated the matter lightly. He occasionally drank freely, but witness never saw him intoxicated. Witness was speaking to deceased a quarter of an hour previous to his death, and he then appeared in his usual health. Dr. Thomas : The deceased was a patient of mine, and was under my care for the last fortnight. He was suffering from fistula, for the cure of which I told him it was necessary that he should undergo an operation ; and to this he readily assented. I prescribed medicine to improve his general health and prepare him for the operation ; and on Saturday last he told me that he had not slept all night, was nervous and frightened at the prospect of being operated on, and was anxious to take chloroform before the operation was performed. Tuesday was the day fixed for this purpose ; and about three o'clock Mr. Barker and I examined the fistula, and before administering the chloroform I asked the deceased particularly if he had ever suffered from any serious illness ; to which he replied in the negative. I also inquired whether he had been subject to cough or palpitation ; and he answered, that some time ago he had suffered slightly from cough. The pulse was good, and Mr. Barker proceeded in the usual manner to administer the chloroform, which shortly produced convulsive twitchings of the muscles. I then went to the door to request the nurse to send up some person to assist in holding the patient in a proper position for the operation, and I returned to the bed and poured a little more chloroform on the handkerchief ; when, it was applied to the face, I observed him splutter at the mouth ; the chloroform was instantly discontinued, but the patient suddenly expired. We tried all the means usually resorted to in cases of suspended animation, but without effect. I had frequently used the same chloroform in other cases. It was not more than a minute after the first application of chloroform that death occurred. About a drachm had been poured on the handkerchief. Dr. Motherwell stated, that he had made a post-mortem examination of the body of the deceased, in the presence of Dr. Howit, Dr. Playne, Dr. Barker, and Dr. Youl. On opening the chest the heart presented an extraordinary appearance. There was considerable serous effusion into the pericardium and the heart itself was larger and more flabby than usual. It was hypertrophied, and there was dilatation of the cavities ; the lungs were healthy, and there was a slight appearance of disease about the liver, such as is observed in persons addicted to intemperance. Where such a state of diseased heart exists death generally supervenes suddenly, and is liable to be caused by any sudden emotion. Death in the present instance was caused by the shock produced by the chloroform, which would not have had such a fatal effect if the heart had been in a healthy state. Unless the attention of a medical man had been particularly directed to the affection of the heart, it would have been very difficult to discover the existence of any such disease. This closed the evidence, and the verdict of the jury was, that the deceased died from the effects of a sudden shock produced by the inhalation of the vapour of chloroform, while suffering under disease of the heart ; but the jury, in recording their verdict, entirely exonerate from blame those medical gentlemen, who directed the administration of a drug which has prevented so much human suffering, and was intended to do so in the present instance.

Discussion

The patient appeared healthy and gave no history of serious illness. Mr. Barker anaesthetized the patient according to the accepted custom : by covering his face with a handkerchief which had been moistened with chloroform. Death occurred almost instantaneously.

According to Lyman (1881), out of 219 deaths which occurred during or following inhalation of chloroform, 15 deaths were at the beginning of the inhalation of the agent ; 99 patients died before complete insensibility ; 70 died during the period of surgery, and the remaining 35 after the completion of surgery.

Lyman also stated that 15 patients died less than two minutes after the start of chloroform anaesthesia out of 52 cases, in which the time between the start of anaesthesia and the occurrence of death was recorded. It seems unlikely that the post–mortem findings were compatible with asymptomatic good health prior to anaesthesia. Perhaps today, more detailed questioning and physical examination would detect preoperatively the abnormal heart.

In conclusion, the following factors, well recognized today, but not at the time, combined to produce the fatal result.
(1) Myocardial disease with pericardial effusion.
(2) Terrified patient with high levels of endogenous catecholamines.
(3) Struggling, coughing patient with rapidly developing hypoxaemia.
(4) Inhalation of unknown concentration of chloroform.
(5) Direct and indirect myocardial depressant effects of chloroform.

It is interesting to postulate that any of today's anaesthetic agents used under the same circumstances might result in a similar outcome.

References

London Medical Gazette (1848): Editorials. 6, 236–239 (Feb. 11)
Lyman, H. M. (1881): Artificial Anaesthesia and Anaesthetics. New York: William Wood and Company, pp.136–201.
Ibid., pp.194–195.
Murray, J. (1873): "Recent views on anaesthetics: their mortality, and mode of administration", London Medical Record, 1, 241–262.

(Reproduced with kind permission from the jarnal *Anaesthesia and Intensive care*.)

Index of Personal Names

【A】
Abbot G. 223, 229
Abe T. 197
Achard E. C. 143
Adriani J. 129, 173
Aiya K. ...... vii, 11, 83, 85, 191
Amano M.
　　...... 35, 59, 61, 171, 182, 183
　　　　199, 200, 201, 202, 204
Aoyagi T. 207
Aoyama T. 45, 123, 161
Araki C. 53, 55, 162
Artusio J. F. 202
Azuma R. 110, 195
Azuma Y. 114

【B】
Bailey P. S. ···51, 53, 55, 161, 197
Baker A. 110
Bernhard von Langenbeck
　　..................... 17, 19
Bier A. 110
Bigelow J. 220
Bigelow H. J. 221
Bleeker 15, 93
Boott F. 220, 225
Braun H. 195

【C】
Chikamori M. 111
Collins V. 217
Czerny V. 17

【D】
Dandy W. 51

【E】
Dohi K. 194
Dye F. C. 202

【E】
Ellis R. H. 214
Emperor Showa 146

【F】
Flexner A. 143
Forbes J. 226
Fraser W. 221
Fujita T. 119
Fukuda T. 173, 200, 201
Furubayashi T. 71
Furukawa K. 183, 204
Furukawa T. 183, 204

【G】
Goto S. 121

【H】
Hanai 75, 76
Hanaoka N. 77
Hanaoka S.
　　...... vii, 9, 63, 77, 83, 190, 207
Hancke H. J. 80
Harvey W. 216
Hayashi S. 172, 178, 198
Higashionna K. 63
Hirata M. 47
Hirota G. 95, 193
Hirota K. 59
Hobson B. 192
Honma G. 192, 193
Hooke R. 5
Horita A. 202
Hoshiko N. 200
Hosoya Y. 195
Hozumi I. 72

Hui–you H. ················ 65, 68

【I】
Ichikawa T. ················ 199
Ichiyanagi Z. ················ 177
Ikeda K. ················ 208
Ikeda S. ················ 29
Imamura R. ················ 193
Inamoto A.
········ 53, 120, 183, 203, 204
Inou–e T. ················ 194
Isashiki D. ················ 66, 67
Isashiki Y. ················ 67
Ishiguro T. ················ 194
Ishihara H. ················ 210
Ito G. ················ 94, 193
Ito H. ················ 110, 195
Itokawa H. ················ 200
Iwai S. ················ 201
Iwanaga B. ················ 77
Iwanaga J. ················ 9, 79
Iwanaga of Kyoto ············ 9
Iwanaga S. ················ 79, 190
Iwanaga S. ················ 79
Iwasaki H. ················ 3
Iwatsuki K.
············ 57, 61, 183, 200, 204

【J】
Jaboulay M. ················ 100
Jackson C. ················ 173
Jacoby ················ 195

【K】
Kagami B. ················ 191
Kamata G. ················ 192
Kato T. ················ 145
Kawanishi Y. ········· 175, 198
Kawasaki D. ················ 193

Kawata S. ················ 201
Ken–tang W. ················ 75
Kimoto S. ········ 175, 198, 201
Kimura K. ················ 110
Kinjo K. ················ 64
Kirshner M. ················ 124
Kitagawa O. ······ 99, 110, 195
Kitamura K. ················ 196
Kitasato S. ················ 142
Kodama Y. ················ 95
Koller C. ················ 105
Kondo T. ············ 123, 195
Kore–eda A. ················ 68
Kusama Y. ············ 167, 198

【L】
Larson M. D. ················ 7
Long C. N. H. ················ 155
Lundy J. S. ············ 45, 49, 197

【M】
Maeda M. ················ 197
Maeda S. ············ 13, 93, 192
Maeda S. ················ 72
Maeda W.
······ 29, 31, 55, 136, 154, 162
199, 201
Mann F. C. ················ 197
Matsui G. ················ 196
Matsuki A. ················ 211
Matsunaga H. ············ 178
Minami S. ············ 139, 196
Miwa Y. ············ 195, 196
Miyakawa J. ················ 191
Miyake G. ················ 192
Miyake H. ··· 43, 121, 141, 146
Miyamoto S. ············ 119, 201
Miyazaki I. ················ 144
Miyazaki R. ················ 193

Mohnike O. G. J.　13, 15, 92, 192
Moolten S.E.　55
Morishima H. O.　59
Morita K.　3
Morton W. T. G.　92, 193, 213, 223
Mukai G.　79
Murayama H.　193
Muto M.　103, 140, 200, 201, 202

【N】
Nagae D.　45, 47, 51, 53, 123, 127, 140, 197
Nagai E.　68
Nagano J.　195
Nagatomi D.　85
Nakagawa K.　196
Nakagawa S.　9, 75, 77, 190
Nakamura M.　201
Nakatani H.　123, 140, 197
Nakayama S.　21, 195
Narabayashi S.　13, 92, 93, 192
Newton I.　5
Ninomiya G.　191
Ninomiya K.　193
Nishimura N.　183, 204

【O】
Obuchi M.　111
Ogata K.　96
Ogata T.　207
Okada W.　194
Okawa S.　201
Omine S.　65
Omori H.　19
Onchi Y.　202

Onishi　75, 76
Ono J.　173
Oyama T.　207, 208

【P】
Pardo C.　100
Park R-S.　25, 114, 129, 197
Perry M. C.　136, 153
Pompe van Meerdervoort　94

【R】
Rienhoff W. F.　51
Robinson J.　213, 214, 220

【S】
Saito M.　23, 25, 55, 114, 197, 198
Saklad M.　3, 29, 103, 135, 153, 155, 158, 165, 167, 172, 198
Sakuragawa Y.　94
Sams C. F.　167, 198
Sato S.　19, 195
Sato S.　97, 194
Sauerbruch F.　124
Schafer P. W.　31
Schaltenbrand G.　161
Schleich C.　194
Schlesinger J.　11, 13, 92, 96, 192
Schreuder　15, 93
Scott W.　221
Scriba J.　17, 106
Sekiguchi S.　41, 118, 196
Shima R.　97, 192
Shimizu K.　33, 55, 161, 162, 165, 197, 198, 200, 201
Shimotsuma K.　113

Shinjo S. C. 87
Shinoi K. 35, 201, 203
Shiota H. 37, 182
Shiozawa S. 201
Shitetsu G. 63
Shizhe W. 63
Shoeki 65
Shojun 65
Shotei 65
Siebold F. von 191
Simpson J. Y. 92, 233, 250
Snow J. 214, 216
Sugimura S. 103
Sugita G. 11
Sugita R. 11, 191
Sugita S. 11, 13, 92, 96, 192
Sykes W. S. 7

【T】
Takahashi T. 183, 204
Takaki K. 21
Takamatsu R. 193
Takamine T. 63, 190
Takashi H. 71, 190
Takashima R. 198
Takemi T. 37, 182
Tamiya T. 162
Tanaka K.
　　..... 51, 55, 123, 140, 162, 197
Tashiro Y. 19
Terada O. 194
Thorek P. 55
Tohyama T. 53
Tongu Y. 195, 196
Torikata R.
　　......... 41, 53, 108, 118, 196
Tovell R. M. 49
Traina V. L. 202
Tsuboi S. 193

Tsuzuki M. 173
Tuo H. 190
Tuohy E. B. 49

【U】
Ueno N. 21, 110, 195
Ume K. 194
Utsuki K. 79

【V】
Vesalius A. 216
Vinci L. Da. 5
Volpitto P. P. 33, 200

【W】
Warren J. C. 223, 229
Wassink 15, 93
Watabe Y. 201
Watanabe J. 195
Watanuki T. 172, 198, 201
Willis W. 95, 193
Wilson L. B. 47

【Y】
Yamamoto T. 201
Yamamura H.
　　... 33, 35, 37, 61, 136, 165, 171
　　182, 183, 186, 199, 200, 201
　　203, 204, 205, 206, 207
Yamanoue O. 190
Yamashita K. 204
Yamato K. 77
Yonezawa T. 183, 204
Yoshida K. 95, 193

【Z】
Zsigmond E. K. .... viii, 213

Index of Subjects

2nd Asian Australasian Congress of Anaesthesiologits 205
50th Annual Meeting of the JSA 210
6110th United States Air Force Hospital 202

【A】
Alcuronium 205, 206
American Journal of Dental Science 220
American Nobel Prize laureates 142
Analects of Confucius, the ... 144
Anesthesia 35, 37
Anesthesia and Reanimation ... 206
Anesthesia Chart 248
Anesthesia Conference 200
Anesthesia Day 209
anesthesia group
.... 165, 166, 199
Anesthesia Terminology 208
Anesthesiology (Masuigaku)
.... 201, 202
Anesthetic Management of Endocrine Disease 207
Anesthetic Method (Masuiho) ... 198
Anglo–Japanese Alliance ... 145
Archives of Clinical Surgery ... 19
Archives of the JSA 211
Army Medical School 45
Asian Australasian Congress of Anaesthesiologists 37
Ateru Kyuho Shiken Setsu 193

Ateru Kyuho Shisetsu ... 13, 192

【B】
baricity 110
Batavia 15, 92
bilzenkruid 81
Birusen 80
Black Battle Ships 136, 137
Blank 20 Years, the
.... 3, 41, 43, 118, 135
board certified anesthesiologists
.... 37, 59, 182, 184, 211
Board on Medical Service System
.... 179
Boshin War 95
Bupivacaine 206

【C】
carbolonium 204
Cardiovascular Anesthesia ... 209
cerebrospinal fluid pressure
.... 111
Charité Hospital 124
Chishi Geka Soron 105
chloroform analgesia
.... 13, 93, 192
chloroform anesthesia
.... 13, 192, 193
cisternal injections 113
cisternal magna 111
cisternal puncture 115
Clinical Anesthesiology (Rinsho masuigaku) 201
closed circle system 135
CO_2 absorption system 135
Colloquium on Anesthesia ... 202
Committee on Board Qualification 204
concept of "Anesthesia" ... 140

Conduction Anesthesia (Dentatsu masuiho) 196
Controversy on Thoracotomy 141
convicts 115
Council of Medical Service System 180
crush syndrome 140, 196
Cyclopropane 135, 200

【D】
Datura 9
Datura alba Nees 85, 190
De humani corporis fabrica 216
De Motu Cordis 216
death caused by spinal anesthesia 196
Deaths due to spinal anesthesia 110
Dejima 13, 92
Delivery and Anesthesia 204
Department of Anesthesiology 163
Desflurane 211
Dialogue with Mohnike, A 13, 93
Droperidol 207
d–Tubocurarine 201
Dutch East India Company factory 13, 15
Dutch East India Factory 92

【E】
electroencephalograph 162, 200
Encyclopedia of Medicine 144
endotracheal anesthesia 135
Endotracheal Anesthesia and Its Precautions (Kikan–nai masuiho oyobi sono chuiten) 201

enflurane 208
enflurane anesthesia 207
epidural opioid therapy 99
ether anaesthesia 220
ether anesthesia 13
ether inhalation 192
ethylene 126
evipan sodium 125

【F】
Far East Journal of Anesthesia, The 202
Fatal Case of Chloroform Anaeshtesia 250
Fatal Case of Chloroform Anesthesia 232, 233
Fellows 211
Fellows of the JSA 183
fentanyl 207
fifth WCA, the 39
First Lines of the Practice of Surgery in the West 192
flexible gastroscopy 125
Fluid Volume Monitoring with Glucose Dilution 210

【G】
Gallamine 206
Gamma Hydroxybutyrate 206
Gassuido School 96
Geishu Domain 95
Geka 51, 198
Geka Hokan 53
Geka Kihai 192
Geka Kihai Zufu 192
Gemayaku 75
general anesthesia 41, 103
General Headquarters of the Allied Powers (GHQ) 27

General Therapeutics, General Anesthesia, Local Anesthesia, Anti–sepsis and Asepsis ······ 196
generally approved designations ············· 59, 179, 180, 182
German Society of Surgery ·································· 19
Gi Family's Genealogy ······· 64
Gisei Kafu ······················ 64, 69
Great Japan Medical Association················· 142
Gripsholm ····················· 161
Gross Clinic ··················· 193
Gun–idan Zasshi················ 49
Gunjin Geka Shinron ········· 107

【H】
halothane ····················· 203
Hexocarbacholine············ 204
historical approach ······ 7, 213
Homestead····················· 161
Honetsugi Ryoji Chohoki ················· 71, 73, 76, 190
hyperbaric solution ···················· 23, 130, 197
hyperbaricity ················· 132
hypobaric solution ··· 23, 124

【I】
Igaku Doshimon ················ 73
Immigration Act of 1924 ··· 146
independent department of anesthesiology ·············· 33, 153, 165, 200
Institute on Anesthesia ······· 200
International Factors ······ 145
intractable trigeminal neuralgia ·································· 99

intradurale Sacralanästhesie ·································· 130
intra–tracheal narcosis ······ 176
intra–tracheal Narkose······ 177
isoflurane ··············· 208, 209

【J】
Jacoby's line ·················· 195
Japan Medical Association ············· 37, 142, 181, 194
Japan Society for Clinical Anesthesia ················· 120
Japan Society for Geriatric Anesthesia ················· 209
Japan Society of Anesthesiology ········ 35, 137, 140, 153, 169 181, 201
Japan Society of Local Anesthesia ················· 208
Japan Surgical Association ·································· 114
Japan Surgical Society (JSS) ············· 17, 139, 170, 194
Japanese Anesthesia History Association··················· 211
Japanese Anesthesia Journals' Review························ 208
Japanese Association for Thoracic Surgery ··· 35, 170
Japanese Association of Medical Sciences ········· 142, 185, 203
Japanese Embassy in Washington, D.C. ·········· 45
Japanese medical community ·································· 142
Japanese Medical Specialty Board ····················· 183
Japanese medical system ··· 27

Japanese Museum of
    Anesthesiology ...... vii, 211
Japanese Society of
    Anesthesiologists (JSA)
    .... vii, 1, 136, 209
Japanese Society of
    Reanimatology 208
Japanese Society of Regional
    Anesthesia 211
Japanese students 15
Japanese United Association of
    Medical Sciences 185
Japanese–American Joint
    Conference on Medical
    Education 103, 153, 198
Jefferson Medical College... 173
Johns Hopkins Hospital ... 197
Johns Hopkins University
    Hospital 51
Joint Research Group on Anesthesia
    200
Joka Sentei 9, 77
Journal of Anesthesia ... 59, 208
*Journal of Anesthesia
    Clinical Report (online)* ... 211
*Journal of the Japan Society for
    Clinical Anesthesia, the* 208
*Journal of the Japan Society of Pain
    Clinicians* 209
JSA annual report 206
JSA Board Certified
    Anesthesiologists 183
JSA Matsuki Prize............ 211
JSA Qualified Anesthesiologists
    183
JSA Research Incentive Prize
    209
JSA Seishu Prize 210
JSA Social Prize................ 209

【K】
Kagoshima Domain 93
Kaitai Shinsho................. 11
Kinsei Kyokusho Masui 195
Kishu Domain 83
Komodoji Temple 87
Korean morning glory... 85, 190
Korean–Japanese Joint
    Symposium 207
Kyokusho Masui 194

【L】
laryngoscopy 173
law suit 195
local anesthesia 41, 103
Local Anesthesia (Kyokusho masui)
    195
*Local Anesthesia and General
    Anesthesia (Kyokusho masuiho
    oyobi zenshin masuiho)*...... 198
Lokalanästhesie 195
London Medical Gazette......... 214
low spinal anesthesia 129
lung surgery 173
Lyon medical 100

【M】
Mafutsusan ... 11, 85, 90, 191
Man–yu zakki 85
Masui 11, 181, 192, 200
masui–gaku 136
masuika–gaku 136
Masuisan...................... 191
Masuikagaku 209
Mayaku 75
Mayaku Ko 76, 80, 190
Mayo Clinic, the
    .... 47, 126, 127, 197

Index of Subjects 261

mechanism of excitement ·········· 197
Medical Center in Washington, D.C. ········· 47
Medical Ethics Committee ·········· 37
Medical Ethics Council ·········· 181, 203
Medical Service Law ········· 180
Meiji Constitution ············ 17
Meiji Government ········· 3, 63
Meiji Restoration, the ······ 41
Methods of Local Anesthesia (Kyokusho mahiho) ········· 196
Methoxyflurane············· 205
Ministry of Education ·········· 143, 163
Ministry of Health and Welfare ·········· 143
modern American anesthesiology ·········· 51
Mona Lisa ····················· 5
mortality rate ················ 122
Morton's Ether Anesthesia ·········· 223
Morton's Public demonstration ·········· 194
Most Recent Anesthesia, the (Saishin masuigaku) ······ 200

Most Recent Surgery and Anesthsia, the (Mottomo atarashii geka to masui) ····················· 199
Mutsu Shujutsu ············ 195
Mutsu to Masui ············ 205

【N】
naso–tracheal intubation ··· 126
national factors ············· 139

National Medical Service Law ·········· 143, 180
Naval Reduction Conferences ·········· 146
Netherlands, the ············ 11
Neurology Institute ········· 162
New Introduction to Anesthesia (Atarashii masuigaku nyumon) ·········· 200
New Local Anesthesia (Shinsen Kyokusho Masui) ············ 197
Newest Surgery and Anesthesia, the ·········· 154
Newsletter of the JSA ········· 209
Nihon Ifu ····················· 79
Nihon Masuika Gakkai··· 136, 209
Nitrous Oxide Seminar ········· 202
Nobel Prize laureates ······ 147
Nyugan Chiken Roku ······ 11, 87

【O】
On the Inhalation of the Vapour of Ether in Surgical Operations ················ 216
Orizuru ······················· 201
Over den Invloed der Inademing van den Zwavel–Aether op Menschen en Dieren ····················· 13

【P】
Pacific War ········· 23, 25, 45, 55, 135, 179
Pain Clinic ············· 205, 208
Painless Delivery (Mutsubunben Kenkyukai) ···204
Pan–Asianism ············· 143
Pancuronium ················· 207
poppies ····················· 190

positive–pressure ventilation ·············· 41, 108
postoperative mortality ······ 141
postoperative mortality rates ·············· 43
Practice of Inhalation Anesthesia, A (Kyunyu masui no jissai) ··· 201
pulse–oximeter ············· 207

【Q】
qualification system ········ 179
Qualified Anesthesiologists ·············· 211
Quincke's puncture ········ 100
Quincke's spinal puncture ·············· 194

【R】
Reconsideration of Anesthesia (Masui no hansei) ········ 202
regional block ············· 129
registered anesthesiologists ·············· 181, 182
Research Society for Pediatric Anesthesia *(Shonimasui kenkyukai)* ············· 207
Research Society of the Pain Clinic ···················· 206
Revista Médica de Chile ····· 100
Rhode Island Hospital ················ 29, 153, 167
Rinsho Masui (Clinical Anesthesia) ·············· 207
Rocuronium ············· 210
Rongo Shusetsu ············· 144
Russo–Japanese War ······ 17
Ryo Nyugan Ki ············· 191
Ryukyu Islands ············· 65
Ryukyu Kingdom ············· 65

【S】
Sacral and Lumbar Anesthesia (Senkotsu oyobi yozui masuiho) ·············· 195
saddle block ················ 129
saddle block technique······ 198
Satsuma Domain ············ 66
Schmerzlose Operationen ······ 194
Sei–i Ryakuron ············· 192
Seikotsu Han ················ 191
Seikotsu Mayaku ··· 74, 190, 191
Seikotsu Shinsho ············· 191
Seishu Hanaoka and His Medicine ·············· 211
semi–official journal ········ 202
Sendai Historical Museum··· 68
sevoflurane ················ 209
Shimazu Domain ············ 66
Shinsen Hiho (A Taoistic Secret) ·············· 68
Shiyi Dexiao Fang ············ 75
Shokokuji Temple············ 95
Short History of Anesthesia in Japan, A ···················· 211
shoulders of giants ············· 5
Shunrinken ················ 89
Simpang Hospital, the ······ 15
Sino–Japanese War ········ 17
social status of anesthesiologists ········ 59
Société de Chirurgie de Lyon ·············· 100
societies of anesthesia ······ 169
Sousan ···················· 74
specially approved designation ··· 59, 153, 179, 180, 182, 204
specially approved specialty ·············· 203
spinal anesthesia ············ 110

spinal morphine ············ 99
spinal opioids ················ 99
spinal terminal sac anesthesia ··· 132
spinocaine ················· 125
status thymico-lymphaticus
　　···································· 196
Surgical Operations and Anesthesia
　　(*Shujutsu to masui*)
　　····························· 158, 199
Sustained Standards of German
　　Medicine ·············· 147
Sykes' phrases ··············· 7

【T】
Taoistic Secret, A ········· 68, 69
Taubman Health Sciences
　　Library ················· 213
terminal sac anesthesia
　　························· 129, 132
textbooks on anesthesia ··· 23
thiamylal sodium ············ 200
thiopental ············ 135, 200
thoracotomy
　　········· 41, 108, 118, 120, 196
thymicolymphatic diatheses
　　···································· 115
Tokyo Society of Anesthesiologists
　　··············· 37, 182, 201, 203
Tokyo Surgical Society ······ 199
Tokyo Surgical Society
　　Conference ············· 166
tracheal anesthesia
　　························· 21, 51, 172

【U】
Unitarian Service Committee
　　········· 27, 167, 198, 200, 202
Unitarian Service Committee
　　Medical Mission ············ 3

【V】
Vecuronium ················ 208

【W】
WCA ·························· 37
Wohlgemuth's apparatus ··· 195
Wood Library–Museum of
　　Anesthesiology ············ 217
World Federation of Societies of
　　Anaesthesiologists ······ 204
World War I ················ 145

【Y】
Yamamura Prize ············ 208
Yangke Zhengchi Zhuosheng
　　······························· 75, 76
Yoka Hiroku ················· 192

【Z】
Zeitschrift für gesamte Medicin
　　···································· 218
Zenshin Masui ················ 194
Zoku Kimpo Roku ········· 80, 81
Zoku Yoka Hiroku ············ 193

By the Same Author

Seishu Hanaoka and His Medicine
-A Japanese Pioneer of Anesthesia and Surgery-

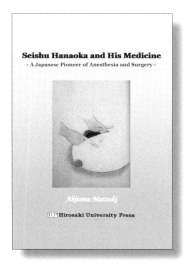

1. Seishu Hanaoka in The Medical History of Japan
2. Seishu Hanaoka and His Family
3. Development of The Anesthetic Mafutsusan
4. The First General Anesthesia for Breast Cancer
5. The Mysteries Surrounding "The Case Report"
6. The List of Breast Cancer Patients
7. Seishu's Surgery and Patient Care
8. The Introduction of Mafutsusan
9. Seishu's School of Shunrinken and Medical Education
10. Seishu's Writings and His Medical Philosophy
11. A Review of The Monographs and Papers on Seishu

ISBN 978-4-902774-68-9
Hardcover 235×155 200pp.
September 2011 2d edition 3,300yen

A Short History of Anesthesia in Japan

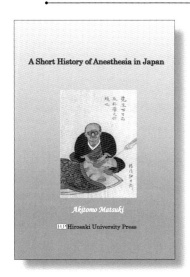

1. Five Important Events during The 200 - Year History of Aesthesiology in Japan
2. Seishū Hanaoka and His Medicine
3. Introduction of Inhaled and Local Anesthesia in Japan
4. Introduction of German Surgery and Foundation of The Japan Surgical Society
5. Establishment of The Academic Society and Independent Departments
6. Japanese Anesthesiology and Developments in Related Academic Societies

Appendix. Chronology of the History of Anesthesia in Japan

ISBN 978-4-902774-93-1
Hardcover 235×155 228pp.
October 2013 4,000yen

The Origin and Evolution of
Anesthesia in Japan

2017年　1月8日　初版第1刷発行

著者　松木明知 (まつき あきとも)

発行所　弘前大学出版会
〒036-8560　青森県弘前市文京町1　HUP
Tel.0172-39-3168　Fax.0172-39-3171

印刷所　やまと印刷株式会社

ISBN978-4-907192-42-6